肺 外 结 核

Extrapulmonary Tuberculosis

[土] 阿尔珀·塞内尔
[土] 哈坎·埃德姆　主编
陆霓虹　杜映荣　郭述良　主译

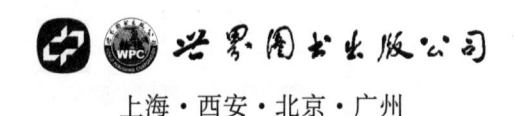

世界图书出版公司
上海·西安·北京·广州

图书在版编目(CIP)数据

肺外结核／(土)阿尔珀·塞内尔,(土)哈坎·埃德姆主编；陆霓虹,杜映荣,郭述良译. —上海：上海世界图书出版公司,2021.8
 ISBN 978-7-5192-8603-3

Ⅰ.①肺… Ⅱ.①阿…②哈…③陆…④杜…⑤郭… Ⅲ.①结核病-诊疗 Ⅳ.①R52

中国版本图书馆CIP数据核字(2021)第108686号

First published in English under the title
Extrapulmonary Tuberculosis
edited by Alper Sener and Hakan Erdem
Copyright © SPRINGER NATURE Switzerland AG, 2019
This edition has been translated and published under licence from
Springer Nature Switzerland AG.

书　　名	肺外结核 Fei Wai Jiehe
主　　编	[土]阿尔珀·塞内尔　[土]哈坎·埃德姆
主　　译	陆霓虹　杜映荣　郭述良
责任编辑	芮晴舟
出版发行	上海世界图书出版公司
地　　址	上海市广中路88号9-10楼
邮　　编	200083
网　　址	http://www.wpcsh.com
经　　销	新华书店
印　　刷	上海天地海设计印刷有限公司
开　　本	787mm×1092mm　1/16
印　　张	13.5
字　　数	220千字
印　　数	1-2000
版　　次	2021年8月第1版　2021年8月第1次印刷
版权登记	图字09-2020-928号
书　　号	ISBN 978-7-5192-8603-3/R·592
定　　价	230.00元

版权所有　翻印必究
如发现印装质量问题,请与印刷厂联系
(质检科电话：021-64366274)

译者名单

主　译

陆霓虹　杜映荣　郭述良

副主译

董昭兴　刘洪璐　杨永锐　吴　磊　李江蕾

李一诗　李晓非

译　者(按姓氏笔画排序)

丁　敏　方如意　白劲松　刘贵明　孙娅萍　李　杰

杨　丽　杨　艳　沈凌筠　陈杨君　欧阳兵　罗　壮

金　媛　高建鹏　黄红丽

编者名单

久姆胡尔·阿尔图克(Cumhur Artuk)：土耳其,安卡拉,卫生科学大学,古尔汉医学院,传染病和临床微生物学系

哈利勒·法提赫·阿斯根(Halil Fatih Aşgün)：土耳其,恰纳卡莱,卡纳卡莱昂塞基兹马特大学,心血管外科

雅库普·哈坎·巴沙兰(Yakup Hakan Basaran)：土耳其,伊斯坦布尔,伊斯坦布尔什姆拉尼耶脑科医院

艾塞·巴蒂雷尔(Ayse Batirel)：土耳其,伊斯坦布尔,卫生科学大学,卡塔尔·卢特菲·基尔达尔博士教育和研究医院,传染病和临床微生物学系

特鲁尔斯·埃里克·比约克朗德·约翰森(Truls Erik Bjerklund Johansen)：挪威,奥斯陆,奥斯陆大学医院泌尿外科和临床医学研究所；丹麦,奥胡斯大学临床医学研究所

阿尔祖·塔斯基兰·科梅兹(Arzu Taskiran Comez)：土耳其,卡纳卡莱,昂塞基兹马特大学医学院,眼科

索菲娅·德·萨拉姆(Sophia De Saram)：英国,伦敦,帝国理工学院,感染与免疫学系

居尔登·厄尔茨(Gülden Ersöz)：土耳其,梅尔辛,梅尔辛大学医学院,传染病和临床微生物学系

乔恩·S. 弗里德兰(Jon S. Friedland)：英国,伦敦,伦敦大学圣乔治分校,感染与免疫研究所

汉尼菲·杰姆·居尔(Hanefi Cem Gul)：土耳其,安卡拉,安卡拉卫生科学大学,古尔汉医学院,传染病和临床微生物学系

巴林·基里尔马兹(Bahadır Kırılmaz)：土耳其,卡纳卡莱,昂塞基兹马特大学,心脏病学系

叶卡捷琳娜·库卡维尼亚(Ekaterina Kulchavenya)：俄罗斯联邦，新西伯利亚结核病研究所；俄罗斯联邦，新西伯利亚，新西伯利亚州立医科大学

齐亚德·A.密目(Ziad A. Memish)：沙特阿拉伯，利雅得，阿尔费萨尔大学医学院卫生部；美国，佐治亚州，亚特兰大，埃默里大学，罗林斯公共卫生学院，休伯特全球卫生部

萨马拉·A.密目(Samara A. Mimesh)：沙特阿拉伯，利雅得阿尔达拉医院和医疗中心

格伊尔·穆里奇-奥斯马尼(Gjyle Mulliqi-Osmani)：科索沃，普里什蒂纳，普里什蒂纳大学医学学院和科索沃普里什蒂纳国家公共卫生研究所

库尔特·G.纳贝尔(Kurt G. Naber)：德国，慕尼黑，慕尼黑工业大学泌尿学系

奈菲斯·奥托普拉克(Nefise Öztoprak)：土耳其，安塔利亚卫生科学大学，安塔利亚培训和研究医院，传染病和临床微生物科

德里亚·奥斯杜克-恩金(Derya Ozturk-Engin)：土耳其，伊斯坦布尔，法提赫苏丹迈赫迈特训练研究医院，传染病和临床微生物学系

科尔内留·彼得鲁·波佩斯库(Corneliu Petru Popescu)：罗马尼亚，布加勒斯特，卡罗尔·达维拉医科大学；维克托·贝布斯传染病和热带病临床医院

露尔·拉卡(Lul Raka)：科索沃，普里什蒂纳，普里什蒂纳大学医学院"哈桑-普里什蒂纳"和科索沃国家公共卫生研究所

盖达·艾哈迈德·谢哈塔(Ghaydaa Ahmed Shehata)：埃及，阿苏特，阿苏特大学

琼·保罗·斯塔尔(Jean Paul Stahl)：法国，格勒诺布尔，阿尔卑斯大学传染病科；塞内加尔，达喀尔，欧洲脑感染研究小组

许利亚·松古尔泰金(Hulya Sungurtekin)：土耳其；德尼兹利，帕穆卡莱大学医学院，麻醉学系

内克拉·埃伦·图莱克(Necla Eren Tulek)：土耳其，安卡拉，安卡拉训练研究医院

菲根·萨里德(Figen Sarıgül)：土耳其，安塔利亚，安塔利亚卫生科学大学训练研究医院，传染病和临床微生物学系

中文版序言

结核病是有史以来伴随人类最长的慢性传染病，也是导致死亡人数最多的慢性传染病之一。结核病不仅是医学上的难题，也是严重威胁人类健康的公共卫生问题，造成巨大的社会经济负担。结核病可累及除头发和指甲以外的全身所有脏器或组织，以肺结核最为常见。

肺外结核指结核病变发生在肺以外的淋巴结（除外胸内淋巴结）、胸膜、气管支气管、骨、关节、泌尿生殖系统、消化系统、中枢神经系统等部位，常以病变器官及部位结核病命名。因其感染途径、表现症状不尽相同，诊断方法、检查手段、治疗方法也各不相同，患者的病情易被其他病症所掩盖，不易早期发现和诊断，与肺结核有明显不同。肺外结核若不及时治疗也会导致严重后果甚至危及生命。因此，需要系统、全面地掌握肺外结核的流行病学、发病机理、临床特征、实验室等辅助检查、治疗方法，以实现肺外结核的精准诊疗。然而，令人遗憾的是目前缺乏关于肺外结核的专业书籍，本书的翻译出版填补了这一空缺。

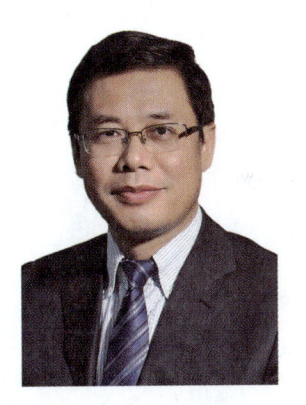

《肺外结核》由陆霓虹、杜映荣等专家主译，以肺外结核为重点，将肺外结核按不同系统分类，计有肺外结核的流行病学、结核性胸膜炎、胃肠结核和结核性腹膜炎、肝胆脾结核、淋巴结结核、结核性关节炎和结核性骨髓炎、结核性脊柱炎、结核性脑膜炎、结核性脑炎、泌尿生殖系统结核、心血管结核、皮肤结核、眼结核、肺外结核的感染控制、重症监护病房中的肺结核等16个章节，全面系统阐述了各肺外结核的流行病学、临床表现、诊断和治疗方法。书籍原版各章均由国际结核病领域著名或知名专家撰写，相信此书

中文版的翻译出版一定会对我国医务工作者诊疗控制肺外结核大有裨益，成为肺外结核诊疗的重要参考书籍。

2021年5月

目 录

1 肺外结核的流行病学 ·· 1
2 结核性胸膜炎 ··· 16
3 胃肠结核和结核性腹膜炎 ·· 26
4 肝胆脾结核 ··· 44
5 淋巴结结核 ··· 60
6 结核性关节炎和结核性骨髓炎 ···································· 72
7 结核性脊椎炎 ··· 84
8 结核性脑膜炎 ·· 102
9 结核性脑炎 ·· 124
10 脊柱结核 ··· 135
11 泌尿生殖系统结核 ·· 143
12 心血管结核 ··· 156
13 皮肤结核 ··· 176
14 眼结核 ··· 182
15 肺外结核的感染控制 ·· 190
16 重症监护病房中的肺结核 ······································ 195
索引 ·· 201

1
肺外结核的流行病学

叶卡捷琳娜·库卡维尼亚,库尔特·G. 纳贝尔和
特鲁尔斯·埃里克·比约克朗德·约翰森

1.1 前言

结核病(tuberculosis,TB)是世界上最致命的传染病之一,被认为是一个主要的全球健康问题。2012 年,约有 860 万人患结核病,其中 130 万人死于该疾病(包括 32 万 HIV 阳性者死亡)。2013 年,约有 900 万人患结核病,其中 150 万人死于该疾病(包括 36 万人 HIV 阳性者死亡)。到 2014 年,全球估计有 960 万人患结核病(男性 540 万、女性 320 万、儿童 100 万),其中 150 万人死于该疾病(包括 40 万人 HIV 阳性者死亡),12% 为 HIV 阳性患者。总结前述数据,我们发现从 2012 年到 2014 年短短 2 年的时间,结核病患者增加了 100 万,死亡人数增加了 20 万[1-4],基于大多数结核病是可以预防的,上述数据是非常可怕的。

结核病可累及全身各个系统,其表现形式多种多样。它可以影响除头发和指甲外的任何器官或组织。世界卫生组织已经认识到结核病是一个全球性问题,特别是肺结核(pulmonary tuberculosis,PTB)。解决结核病这一全球性问题,不仅在医学上具有重大意义,更具有重大的社会意义,因为肺外结核(extrapulmonary tuberculosis,EPTB)是男女不育最常见的原因之一,特别是在结核流行地区,结核病的性传播途径也被一些研究所报道[5-7]。

1.2 肺外结核的流行病学

在过去的几十年里,肺外结核的发病率不断增加,现有的观点认为主要是由于 HIV 发病率和器官移植数量的逐年增加导致的[8,9]。尽管现在

EPTB 的发病率低于 PTB,并且是国家结核病控制项目的次要指标,但在艾滋病流行期间,其重要性在全球范围内有所增加[10]。EPTB 的发病率根据地域、伴随疾病、主要症状、流行病史、时期等因素的影响而变化。在韩国,EPTB 最常见的感染部位是胸膜,其次是淋巴结,胃肠器官、骨骼和关节、中枢神经系统和泌尿生殖系统结核很少累及[11]。

在孟加拉国,EPTB 约占结核病患者所有病例的 15%～20%,在社会经济地位低的群体中更为常见,约占 60%。在 16～45 岁年龄组(平均年龄 35.67±14.6 岁)群体中,EPTB 的发病率高达 55%,其中女性患者较多,约占 60%[12]。在巴西,HIV 的感染率从 1981 年的 6.8 人/10 万人上升到 1991 年的 7.0 人/10 万人。PTB 的病例数从 2001 年到 2009 年减少了 23.7%,但 EPTB 病例数仅减少了 5.9%[10]。在印度,EPTB 占结核病病例的 15%～20%,对 2 219 例 EPTB 患者进行治疗后结果发现,15～45 岁年龄组的患者中男性患者较为多见,EPTB 患者的总体治疗完成率为 84%,其中 HIV 阳性患者的治疗完成率仅为 66%,而 HIV 阴性 EPTB 患者的治疗完成率高达 86%。根据累及部位的不同,观察到的治疗完成率如下:淋巴结结核 90.9%,泌尿生殖系统结核(UGTB)92.6%,骨和关节结核 86%,结核性胸腔积液 84.7%,腹部结核 76%,中枢神经系统结核(结核瘤和脑膜炎)63.7%。其中 173 例(7.8%)患者未记录 EPTB 的累及部位[13]。

在大多数情况下,EPTB 常发生在免疫抑制的患者中,作为血源性传播引起的严重疾病之一。在一些地区,作者发现 EPTB 常累及腹部器官和泌尿生殖系统,而中枢神经系统和骨骼肌肉系统少见。常用 CT 检测各种 EPTB 的累及情况,但中枢神经系统和骨骼肌肌肉系统以 MRI 检查为金标准进行评估。很多患者由于临床症状不典型,确诊往往被延误[14]。

在美国 1993 年至 2006 年报告的 253 299 例病例中,73.6% 为 PTB,18.7% 为 EPTB,根据累及部位的不同,EPTB 分为淋巴(40.4%)、胸膜(19.8%)、骨和(或)关节(11.3%)、泌尿生殖系统(6.5%)、脑膜(5.4%)、腹膜(4.9%)和未分类的 EPTB(11.8%)。与 PTB 相比,EPTB 易感性与女性性别和外国出生有关,但与 HIV 阳性与否几乎同等相关,与多药耐药性和一系列结核病危险因素负相关,特别是与无家可归和过量饮酒的群体相关[15]。

在巴西,总共 427 548 例 TB 病例中,有 57 217 例(13.4%)为耐多药结核,13 989 例(3.3%)为 PTB 并发 EPTB。EPTB 患者中白种人占 16.7%,且 29.1% 的患者接受过 5～8 年的教育。在伴随疾病中,HIV 患者是数量最多的,酗酒、糖尿病和精神疾病等危险因素与 PTB 有关,但与 EPTB 无关[10]。

巴西关于 EPTB 的累及情况如图 1-1 所示。

在巴西,尽管 EPTB 患者主要是成人群体,但仍有高达 1/4 的 EPTB 病例发生在 14 岁以下的儿童中[10]。

为了进行比较,我们在统计了西伯利亚 1999 年至 2011 年 EPTB 的累及情况(图 1-2)[16]。2011 年,泌尿男性生殖系统结核的患者比率较前几年下降,但骨和关节结核的患者比率上升,两者都约占 EPTB 的 1/3。肺结核是孟加拉国非常常见的疾病。通过对 216 例活检标本进行回顾性组织病理

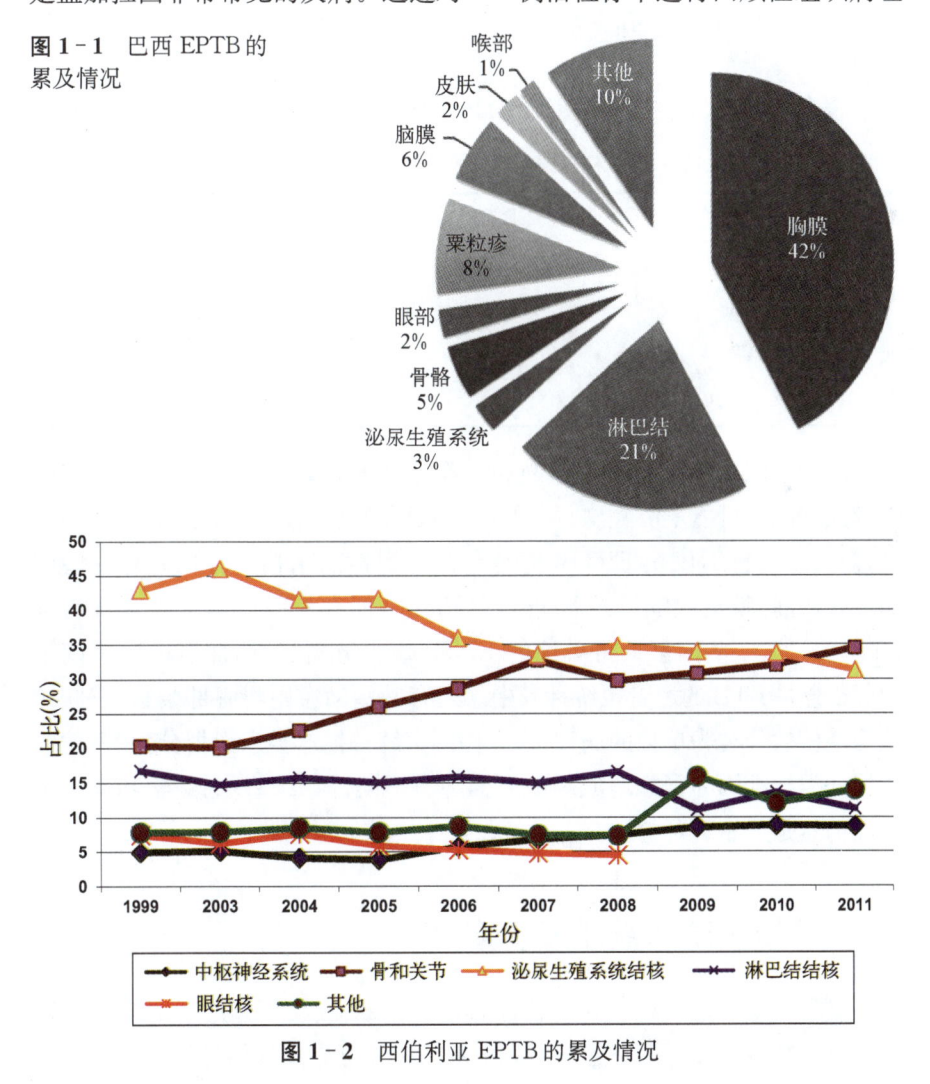

图 1-1 巴西 EPTB 的累及情况

图 1-2 西伯利亚 EPTB 的累及情况

学研究,评估 EPTB 在不同器官中的分布。结果显示女性患者占多数,共有126 例。淋巴结是 EPTB 最常见的部位(62.9%),其次是皮肤和皮下组织(17.59%)、肠(11.11%)、乳房(2.77%)、女性生殖道(2.31%)、男性生殖道(1.38%)以及骨和关节(1.85%)。136 例结核性淋巴结炎中,颈部淋巴结 96 例(70.58%)、腋窝淋巴结 18 例(13.23%)、肠系膜淋巴结 12 例(3.82%)、腹股沟淋巴结 10 例(7.35%)。颈部淋巴结是 EPTB 非常常见的部位[17]。

在波兰 2013 年登记的所有结核病患者中,有 415 名患者被诊断为 EPTB,占所有登记病例的 5.7%。其中结核性胸膜炎有 142 例,为主要构成部分,其次为外周淋巴结结核 104 例,泌尿生殖系统结核 58 例,骨关节结核 44 例[18]。

表 1-1 显示了在不同国家,EPTB 在所有类型结核病中所占的百分比。

表 1-1 EPTB 在各国结核病中所占的百分比

国　家	EPTB 百分比	来　源
孟加拉国	20	[15]
印　度	15~20	[16]
巴　西	13.4	[7]
波　兰	5.7	[24]

由于不同国家对 EPTB 诊断和分类标准的差异,EPTB 最准确的流行病学数据统计可能不够完整,例如在巴西,粟粒型结核被认为是 EPTB 的一种,而实际上它不仅是 EPTB,更是一种广泛性的结核病。在另外一些国家,结核性胸膜炎和喉结核被分类为 EPTB,而在另一些国家则被认为是 PTB。另外,一些国家只将单纯的 EPTB 作为分类标准,而有的国家则把 EPTB 合并 PTB 的患者也统计其中。还有一些国家则将腹部结核、皮肤结核等结核病分类为单独的病种,也有些国家统一把这类患者划分为"其他"。尽管分类标准因为国家地域等的原因各有不同,但 EPTB 的医学和社会重要性仍然是毋庸置疑的。

1.3　泌尿生殖系统结核(UGTB)

泌尿生殖系统结核(urogenital tuberculosis, UGTB)是指由结核分枝杆菌或牛结核分枝杆菌引起的泌尿生殖系统并可累及其他任何组织和器官的感染性炎症。根据定义,它包括泌尿系统结核及女性生殖系统结核[16,19,20],是最常见EPTB表现形式之一。UGTB是EPTB常见的分类之一,其患病数量位于各类EPTB第四位,来自北美的研究甚至认为UGTB是仅次于结核性胸膜炎和淋巴结核的第三种最常见的EPTB[22],但由于其起病隐匿,临床表现特异性低等原因,在临床上,往往容易被临床医师漏诊[21]。

从原发肺部结核病灶开始,2%~20%的患者可通过血行播散到肾、前列腺和附睾,再通过输尿管下行播散到膀胱和尿道,然后再通过输精管感染内外生殖器,从而发展为UGTB。在巴西,UGTB可发生在所有年龄段的群体,但其主要集中在40~50岁的中年男性,在其他国家,不同性别、不同年龄段的人群患UGTB的比率可能会有所不同[23]。UGTB往往起病隐匿,一般在疾病晚期才会出现临床症状,这常导致UGTB无法在疾病早期得到确诊,从而发生泌尿生殖器官被严重破坏的后果。菲格雷多(Figueiredo)等人的报道称肾功能衰竭往往是UGTB患者最初的临床表现,尽管肾内科医师、泌尿科医师和传染病专家早已认识到这种情况,但其他内科医师对UGTB仍知之甚少[23]。

在抗菌药物出现之前,UGTB的患病率更高,泌尿外科的住院患者约有1/5为UGTB的患者,超过1/3的化脓性肾病是由结核感染引起的,其患者大多为年轻人,男女患病比率无显著差异[23]。现在,UGTB是结核病流行国家中最常见的EPTB类型之一,但在低发病率国家,UGTB较为罕见[22,25]。在发达国家,40%以上的EPTB病例是由泌尿生殖系统结核引起的[26]。在欧洲,对比当地人,UGTB患者在移民群体中更为常见[27]。在大多数的卫生健康中心,肾结核的确诊往往较为困难,它可能是原发结核病播散性传播累及脏器,也可能是一种局部的泌尿生殖系统疾病[8]。对于免疫缺陷和疾病高发区域的患者,当出现不明原因的尿路感染时应警惕该疾病的发生[8]。

UGTB在所有EPTB患者中所占的比率,因为不同国家、不同地区、不同群体、不同时期而有所不同。一些学者认为UGTB是第三种最常见的EPTB类型,占EPTB总病例的15%~20%,甚至有的报告统计数据高达40%[22,25,26],而也有一些学者报告的比率仅为4%~17%[8,25,26]。

在意大利,UGTB约占所有EPTB的27%,其发病原因主要是其他部位结核病灶的继发感染或泌尿生殖系统的原发感染[9]。尽管UGTB是结核病流行国家最常见的EPTB类型之一,但在结核病发病率较低的国家,UGTB所占的比率仍较低[16,19,20]。比如在韩国,UGTB在所有肺外部位中发病率是最低的[11]，据统计，2006—2013年间在韩国确诊的135例肺外结核患者中，只有6例患有UGTB，占比为4.4%[28]。在波兰，415名被诊断为肺外结核的患者中，仅有58名（14.0%）为UGTB[18]。在土耳其，UGTB的占比为5.4%[29]。在孟加拉国，UGTB的比率也很低[12]。不同国家UGTB在EPTB患者中所占的比例如表1-2所示。

表1-2 不同国家UGTB在EPTB患者中所占的比率

国 家	UGTB在EPTB患者中所占的比率	来 源
意大利	27.0	[21]
韩 国	4.4	[23]
波 兰	14.0	[24]
土耳其	5.4	[25]
西伯利亚	22.9～46.0	[26]

由于该疾病起病隐匿、临床表现缺乏特异性等原因，往往容易被临床医师漏诊。因此，关于该病的流行病学统计数据可能存在一定的不准确性[19]。

分析1999年到2015年期间俄罗斯远东联邦地区和西伯利亚的UGTB的发病情况，发现在所有的EPTB病例中，UGTB的比例在2003年最高，为46%，2014年最低，为22.9%。根据门诊病历，UGTB中的肾结核患者中，肾结核Ⅰ期占21.2%～37%，Ⅱ期占26%～53.5%，海绵状溃疡病变期占21.6%～37%，前列腺结核的发病率从2003年的0%，2008年的7.1%到2013年的54.2%逐年增加，平均发病率为33.9%[30]。

目前来看，无法估计俄罗斯东部UGTB的真实发病率。近1/4的UGTB患者在接受医学评估时，都有长达5年甚至更长时间的漏诊误诊现象存在。新技术的引进提高了UGTB的细菌学检出率，使得UGTB病例中前列腺结核的检出率增至35.7%[30]。

在对2009年到2014年1 036例疑似泌尿系统结核（urinary tuberculosis，UTB）患者进行评估后，挑选出193例UTB患者进行流行病学、临床特点和耐药性的统计评估。结果显示，尿路刺激征（61.1%）和腰痛（49.2%）是UTB最常见的症状，出现镜下血尿（63.2%）和蛋白尿（45.6%）的患者比率也较高，尿TB-DNA阳性率为66.3%，培养阳性率为13.1%，涂片阳性率为9.8%。结核分枝杆菌总耐药率为39.7%（至少对1种药物耐药），其中

20.7%为多重耐药(至少同时对利福平和异烟肼产生耐药)。实验室检查是UGTB确诊的关键,对于疑似UGTB的患者,推荐用PCR技术检测结核分枝杆菌代替杆菌培养等方法作为检查结核疑似患者的常规技术手段[31]。

为了估计流行地区儿童和青少年肾结核(kidney tuberculosis, KTB)的患病率,我们回顾了西伯利亚131例UGTB患者和吉尔吉斯斯坦819例UGTB患者的病史[32]。在西伯利亚,只有2名儿童和1名青少年在早期被发现患有UGTB(占UGTB患者的2.3%),均为KTB 1期。在吉尔吉斯斯坦的819例UGTB患者中,也仅有17名儿童和21名青少年(占所有UGTB患者的4.6%),且所有人都有很长的病史并接受过手术干预,其中6人患有瘘管,2名青少年患有微囊虫病,且为膀胱结核4期,所有儿童病例中,只有2名被诊断为KTB 1级,KTB 2级、KTB 3级、KTB 4级的病例数分别为4例、8例、3例。也就是说,高达64.5%的患者是在UGTB晚期和进展期才被诊断出来的[32]。

UGTB的发病原因可分为两种:一种是由其他结核病灶播散性传播导致的继发感染,另一种为泌尿生殖系统的原发感染[8]。结核病的肾受累可能是播散性传播导致的继发感染,也可能是局部泌尿生殖系统的原发病灶[9]。对于免疫缺陷和疾病高发区域的患者,当出现不明原因的尿路感染时医师应警惕该疾病的发生[9]。

有学者指出,慢性肾病患者患结核病的风险会显著增加[33]。两种疾病之间具有一定的联系性已经在40多年前开始就有所报道,但这两种疾病之间具体的相互作用到今天仍然知之甚少,现有的相关文献指出,透析和肾移植患者患结核病的风险似乎更高,但肾结核的易感性也与社会的经济状况、人口水平和患者伴随疾病等因素具有一定的相关性[34-36]。

1.4 淋巴结结核

肉芽肿性疾病,如结核病和结节病等导致淋巴结肿大与转移性淋巴结或淋巴瘤的外观非常相似,常用超声检查作为早期的诊断评估和鉴别手段。淋巴结中的无回声或低回声区域可能代表坏死或转移性出血,但也可能代表发炎或淋巴结中的化脓病灶。诊断为淋巴结异常的患者可采用超声引导下靶向细针穿刺活检或淋巴结切除术,进行组织病理学检查以便明确诊断[37]。

在孟加拉国、印度和土耳其，淋巴结是肺外结核最常见的受累部位，其在所有肺外结核患者中的占比分别为50%、34.4%和39.4%[28]，且在女性患者中更为常见，约占58%[13]。

T-SPOT实验对结核病的诊断价值因感染部位不同而有所差异，对淋巴结结核等慢性结核的敏感性较高，对结核性淋巴结炎诊断的特异性较高。T-SPOT实验的诊断价值因检测的具体方法、种族的不同及淋巴结炎部位的不同而有所差异，该技术更适用于结核病流行地区关于该疾病的诊疗[38]。

1.5 中枢神经系统结核(CNS-TB)

中枢神经系统结核(CNS-TB)是一种具有高病死率的严重结核病[39]，常发生颅内结核性动脉瘤破裂等严重并发症[40]。

CNS-TB常表现为结核性脑膜炎、颅内结核和脊髓蛛网膜炎三种形式。结核性脑膜炎在西方国家较为多见，常表现为亚急性或慢性脑膜炎综合征，前驱症状常表现为全身不适、发热和头痛，进展期常出现神志改变和局灶性神经体征，疾病晚期常出现昏迷嗜睡，患者通常在发病后5~8周内死亡，血管炎常常导致基底节区发生梗死，是发病率和病死率的主要决定因素。中枢神经系统结核通常表现为结核性脑膜炎，结核瘤多见于颅内，较少累及脊髓，颅内结核瘤合并髓内结核瘤更是极为罕见。然而，由于部分颅内结核患者早期常表现为无症状或症状较轻，所以脊髓结核的患者仍应进行脑部MRI的检查以进一步评估病情[41,42]。

根据印度结核病管理协会的统计数据，在印度，每天约有1 000名患者死于CNS-TB，且在青壮年中具有较高的发病率和病死率，是导致印度青壮年劳动力丧失的主要原因[42]。根据其他印度关于结核病的统计报告，CNS-TB约占EPTB患者的9.4%[13,43]。

为评估印度东北部颅内结核患者的临床和影像学表现，研究者采用前瞻性研究的方法分析了93名患者(38.7%的女性和61.3%的男性)的患病情况，结果显示酗酒是该疾病最常见的危险因素，约占19.4%。头痛是其最常见的症状，约占90.3%。合并HIV感染的患者有11例，隐球菌感染有3例，弓形虫感染有2例。脑脊液分析抗酸杆菌涂片阳性者为1例，结核PCR检测和BACTEC结核分枝杆菌培养阳性者分别为1例和3例(BACTEC

MGIT 960 是一种全自动、无放射性的培养系统,能够高效、快速、准确地从临床标本中分离出结核分枝杆菌,被广泛推荐使用)。从影像学表现来看,表现为基底有渗出物、结核球、脑水肿、脑积水、脑梗死和脑脓肿的占比分别为 21.7%、28.6%、27%、32.9%、21%和 2.9%。其中共有 25 名(26.9%)患者死亡,38 名患者(40.9%)出现偏瘫、截瘫、视力丧失和听力损失等神经后遗症[44]。

中枢神经系统受累的结核病在摩洛哥相当罕见,但多灶性或粟粒型肺结核较为常见。评估脑外结核是否合并中枢神经系统感染对并发结核性脑膜病变的患者具有重大意义[45]。

随着多耐药结核患者的逐渐增多,CNS‐TB 的症状变得越来越不典型,病史也变得越来越复杂,常规的血清学试验诊断技术往往耗时较长,很可能会延误治疗,错过最佳诊疗时期。因此,熟悉 CNS‐TB 的各种影像学特征,以确保该疾病的早发现、早诊断、早治疗,从而降低与该病相关的高发病率和病死率是非常重要的。运用 MRI 等影像学检查方法将有助于不典型 CNS‐TB 的诊断[46]。

1.6 骨关节结核

脊柱结核,也被称为波特病,于 1779 年被珀西亚尔·波特(Perciall Pott)首次报道。其起病隐匿,首发症状常表现为背部疼痛和局部压痛,以及与结核病相关的一些全身症状,在疾病发展后期,可出现脊柱后凸畸形和神经压迫症状等临床表现,约占骨关节结核患者数量的 50%～60%,是最常见的肺外结核之一[47]。

结核病是发展中国家主要的健康问题之一。约 1/3 感染结核分枝杆菌的儿童有肺外受累。在印度,脊柱是骨关节结核最常见的受累部位,其发病率约为 1%～6%,股骨、胫骨和腓骨受累也较为常见,无关节受累的单纯性结核性骨髓炎仅占所有骨关节结核病例的 2%～3%。在儿童结核病中,播散性骨骼受累非常罕见,约占 7%,颅骨骨髓炎则更为罕见,仅占 1%[48]。

在美国,骨骼肌肉结核约占所有 EPTB 病例的 10%,是 EPTB 的第三大常见累及部位,仅次于胸膜和淋巴结。脊柱受累(结核性脊柱炎或波特病)约占所有肌肉骨骼结核病例的一半,是最常见的骨骼肌肉结核类型,可能不伴有肺部受累[49]。

在中国,结核病已经变得非常常见。相关统计数据表明,骨关节结核约占 EPTB 病例总数的 10%,其中约 44% 的患者为脊柱结核,脊柱是最常见的受累部位[50]。然而,也有学者的统计结果显示,骨关节结核仅占所有结核病病例的 1%~2%[51]。

在土耳其,约 7.4% 的 EPTB 患者患有骨结核,约 20% 的结核病患者累及肌肉骨骼系统,大部分主要影响脊柱和髋膝关节等大关节,约 10% 的患者会出现手部受累,单纯的手部或手腕结核较为少见[28,52]。

格罗弗(Grover)等人报道了一例较为罕见的骨骼结核病例,其结核感染病灶位于胸骨,临床表现为上腹部肿胀,影像学检查 CT 和 MRI 显示剑突糜烂性骨髓炎,并伴有邻近软组织炎症,在超声引导下穿刺活检,结果显示结核分枝杆菌检测阳性[53]。

1.7 腹部结核

腹部结核早在公元前 4 世纪希波克拉底的著作中就已经有所认识。虽然消化系统结核病并不像肺结核病那么常见,但它仍是结核病相关高发病率和病死率的重要原因。其主要是结核分枝杆菌通过消化道、血源性播散或病灶邻近器官蔓延而传播[54]。40% 的儿童肠道结核可以通过微生物学检验进行确诊[55]。

胃肠道结核常与恶性肿瘤的某些临床表现相似,特别是在老年人患者中。曾经有一位 46 岁女性患者,有 6 个月的腹部间歇性疼痛病史,并伴有低热、体重减轻和食欲下降等临床表现。CT 示回肠末端弥漫性长节段增厚、回盲部交界处、升结肠和结肠脾曲变窄,提示为感染性病灶。结肠镜检查显示脾曲有溃疡结节状病变,增加了结肠癌以及升结肠和盲肠增厚的可能性。活检涂片示少量抗酸杆菌(AFBs),GeneXpert[56]检测结核分枝杆菌阳性。

在美国,腹部结核较为少见,其中约 2%~3% 的患者患有结肠癌。由于三种疾病的临床表现、影像学检查结果和内镜检查极为相似,结肠癌常被误诊为克罗恩病或结肠癌[54]。在印度,腹部结核约占 EPTB 的 12.8%[13]。

对一名无症状的胰周肿块样病变患者进行超声引导下的细针抽吸(EUS-FNA)活检,PCR 结果显示结核分枝杆菌检测阳性。此外,对于有淋巴结肿大的患者,包括腹部淋巴结肿大的患者,应警惕结核性淋巴结炎的发生,其是有可能存在的[58]。

1.8　EPTB 的治疗结果

　　EPTB 在疾病的早期阶段开始治疗疗效是最佳的,对于高度怀疑本病的患者,应尽早开始治疗,无须等待实验室检查结果。四联化疗方案异烟肼＋利福平＋吡嗪酰胺＋乙胺丁醇可以最大限度地发挥抗菌作用,并降低治疗过程中出现耐药性的可能性。除了晚期疾病外,使用激素类药物治疗可以降低该疾病的发病率和病死率[13,49]。但在 HIV 感染患者和 CNS－TB 患者中,EPTB 的治疗效果很差[13]。

　　有研究者通过制备了一种新的纳米载体,使得加替沙星可以更好地通过血脑屏障,从而治疗中枢神经系统结核[59]。

1.9　小结

　　EPTB 可累积全身多个系统,临床表现多种多样,医师对该疾病的正确评估十分重要。当遇到病史复杂、对症治疗效果欠佳的患者应注意排查结核感染。由于各国对 EPTB 的分类各不相同,一些国家只将单纯性的 EPTB 纳入此类,而另一些国家不论是原发还是继发,有无其他系统受累归类为 EPTB,因此 EPTB 具体的分布情况统计较为困难。统计分析 EPTB 及其各亚型的具体分布情况,具有重要的医学和社会意义。

参考文献

[1] WHO Global tuberculosis report 2015: who.int/tb/publications/global_report/en/.
[2] WHO Global tuberculosis report. 2013. http://www.eurosurveillance.org/ViewArticle.aspx? ArticleId=20615.
[3] Tuberculosis. Fact sheet N° 104. Reviewed March 2016. Key facts. who.int/mediacentre/factsheets/fs104/en/.
[4] WHO Fact sheet N°104. Reviewed March 2014, available on http://www.who.int/mediacentre/factsheets/fs104/en/.
[5] Kulchavenya E. Urogenital tuberculosis: epidemiology, diagnosis, therapy. Cham\Heidelberg\New York\Dordrecht\London: Springer; 2014.- 137 p. ISBN 978-2-319-04836-9. https://doi.org/10.1007/978-3-319-04837-6.
[6] Ishrat S, Fatima P. Genital tuberculosis in the infertile women — an update.

Mymensingh Med J. 2015; 24(1): 215-20.
[7] Caliskan E, Cakiroglu Y, Sofuoglu K, Doger E, Akar ME, Ozkan SO. Effects of salpingectomy and antituberculosis treatments on fertility results in patients with genital tuberculosis. Int J Urol. 2014; 21(11): 1177. https://doi.org/10.1111/iju.12581. Epub 2014 Jul 23.
[8] Toccaceli S, Persico Stella L, Diana M, Taccone A, Giuliani G, De Paola L, et al. Renal tuberculosis: a case report. G Chir. 2015; 36(2): 76-78.
[9] Daher Ede F, da Silva GB Jr, Barros EJ. Renal tuberculosis in the modern era. Am J Trop Med Hyg. 2013; 88(1): 54-64. https://doi.org/10.4269/ajtmh.2013.12-0413.
[10] Gomes T, Reis-Santos B, Bertolde A, Johnson JL, Riley LW, Maciel EL. Epidemiology of extrapulmonary tuberculosis in Brazil: a hierarchical model. BMC Infect Dis. 2014; 14(9. Published online 2014 Jan 8) https://doi.org/10.1186/1471-2334-14-9.
[11] Lee JY. Diagnosis and Treatment of Extrapulmonary Tuberculosis. Tuberc Respir Dis. 2015; 78: 47-55.
[12] Quddus MA, Uddin MJ, Bhuiyan MM. Evaluation of extra pulmonary tuberculosis in Bangladeshi patients. Mymensingh Med J. 2014; 23(4): 758-763.
[13] Cherian JJ, Lobo I, Sukhlecha A, Chawan U, Kshirsagar NA, Nair BL, Sawardekar L. Treatment outcome of extrapulmonary tuberculosis under Revised National Tuberculosis Control Programme. Indian J Tuberc. 2017; 64(2): 104-8. https://doi.org/10.1016/j.ijtb.2016.11.028. Epub 2017 Jan 11.
[14] Kienzl-Palma D, Prosch H. Extrathoracic manifestations of tuberculosis. Radiologe. 2016; 56(10): 885-889.
[15] Peto HM, Pratt RH, Harrington TA, LoBue PA, Armstrong LR. Epidemiology of extrapulmonary tuberculosis in the United States, 1993-2006. Clin Infect Dis. 2009; 49(9): 1350-1357. https://doi.org/10.1086/605559.
[16] Kulchavenya E. Epidemiology of urogenital tuberculosis in Siberia. Am J Infect Control. 2013; 41(10): 945-946.
[17] Begum A, Baten MA, Begum Z, Alam MM, Ahsan MM, Ansari NP, et al. A retrospective histopathological study on extra-pulmonary tuberculosis in Mymensingh. Mymensingh Med J. 2017; 26(1): 104-108.
[18] Korzeniewska-Koseła M. Tuberculosis in Poland in 2013. Przegl Epidemiol. 2015; 69(2): 277-282, 389-393.
[19] Kulchavenya E. Extrapulmonary Tuberculosis: are statistical reports accurate? Ther Adv Infect Dis. 2014; 2(2): 61-70. https://doi.org/10.1177/2049936114528173.
[20] Kulchavenya E, Naber K, Bjerklund-Johansen T-E. Urogenital tuberculosis: classification, diagnosis and treatment. Eur Urol Suppl. 2016; 15(4): 112-121.
[21] Fillion A, Koutlidis N, Froissart A, Fantin B. Investigation and management of genitourinary tuberculosis. Rev Med Interne. 2014; 35(12): 808-814. https://doi.org/10.1016/j.revmed.2014.07.006. Epub 2014 Sep 17. Review.
[22] Sourial MW, Brimo F, Horn R, Andonian S. Genitourinary tuberculosis in North America: a rare clinical entity. Can Urol Assoc J. 2015; 9(7-8): E484-489.

https://doi.org/10.5489/cuaj.2643.
[23] Marion G. Traite d'Urologie. Paris: Masson; 1940.
[24] Figueiredo A, Lucon A, Srougi M. Urogenital Tuberculosis. Microbiol Spectr. 2017; 5(1): TNMI7-0015-2016. https://doi.org/10.1128/microbiolspec.TNMI7-0015-2016.
[25] Kumar S, Kashyapi BD, Bapat SS. A rare presentation of tuberculous prostatic abscess in young patient. Int J Surg Case Rep. 2015; 10: 80-82. https://doi.org/10.1016/j.ijscr.2015.03.028. Epub 2015 Mar 18.
[26] Sanches I, Pinto C, Sousa M, Carvalho A, Duarte R, Urinary Tuberculosis PM. Serious complications may occur when diagnosis is delayed. Acta Medica Port. 2015; 28(3): 382-385. Epub 2015 Jun 30.
[27] Lenk S. Genitourinary tuberculosis in Germany: diagnosis and treatment. Urologe. 2011; 50(12): 1619-1627.
[28] Lee HY, Lee J, Lee YS, Kim MY, Lee HK, Lee YM, Shin JH, Ko Y. Drug-resistance pattern of Mycobacterium tuberculosis strains from patients with pulmonary and extrapulmonary tuberculosis during 2006 to 2013 in a Korean tertiary medical center. Korean J Intern Med. 2015; 30(3): 325-334. https://doi.org/10.3904/kjim.2015.30.3.325. Epub 2015 Apr 29.
[29] Sunnetcioglu A, Sunnetcioglu M, Binici I, Baran AI, Karahocagil MK, Saydan MR. Comparative analysis of pulmonary and extrapulmonary tuberculosis of 411 cases. Ann Clin Microbiol Antimicrob. 2015; 14: 34. https://doi.org/10.1186/s12941-015-0092-2.
[30] Shevchenko SY, Kulchavenya EV, Alekseeva TV. The epidemiological situation of urogenital tuberculosis in Siberia and the Far East. Urologiia. 2016; (6): 65-70.
[31] Ye Y, Hu X, Shi Y, Zhou J, Zhou Y, Song X, et al. Clinical Features and Drug-Resistance Profile of Urinary Tuberculosis in South-Western China: A Cross-sectional Study. Medicine (Baltimore). 2016; 95(19): e3537. https://doi.org/10.1097/MD.0000000000003537.
[32] Kulchavenya E, Mukanbaev K. Urogenital tuberculosis in children and teenagers in epidemic region. Eur Urol Suppl. 2014; 13: e667.
[33] Ostermann M, Palchaudhuri P, Riding A, Begum P, Milburn HJ. Incidence of tuberculosis is high in chronic kidney disease patients in South East England and drug resistance common. Ren Fail. 2016; 38(2): 256-261. https://doi.org/10.3109/0886022X.2015.1128290. Epub 2016 Jan 4.
[34] Romanowski K, Clark EG, Levin A, Cook VJ, Johnston JC. Tuberculosis and chronic kidney disease: an emerging global syndemic. Kidney Int. 2016. pii: S0085-2538(16)30053-9; 90 https://doi.org/10.1016/j.kint.2016.01.034.
[35] Sutariya HC, Panchal TN, Pandya VK, Patel KN. Disseminated tuberculosis involving allogra ft in a renal transplant recipient. J Glob Infect Dis. 2016; 8(1): 55-56. https://doi.org/10.4103/0974-777X.176151.
[36] Shibata S, Shono E, Nishimagi E, Yamaura K. A patient with urinary tract tuberculosis during treatment with etanercept. Am J Case Rep. 2015; 16: 341-346. https://doi.org/10.12659/AJCR.893416.
[37] Białek EJ, Jakubowski W. Mistakes in ultrasound diagnosis of superficial lymph

nodes. J Ultrason. 2017; 17(68): 59-65. https://doi.org/10.15557/JoU.2017.0008. Epub 2017 Mar 31.

[38] Liu Q, Li W, Chen Y, Du X, Wang C, Liang B, et al. Performance of interferon-γ release assay in the diagnosis of tuberculous lymphadenitis: a meta-analysis. Peer J. 2017; 5: e3136. https://doi.org/10.7717/peerj.3136.eCollection 2017.

[39] Francisco NM, Hsu NJ, Keeton R, Randall P, Sebesho B, Allie N, et al. TNF-dependent regulation and activation of innate immune cells are essential for host protection against cerebral tuberculosis. J Neuroinflammation. 2015; 12(1): 125. Epub ahead of print.

[40] Mani SSR, Mathansingh AJ, Kaur H, Iyyadurai R. Ruptured intracranial tuberculous aneurysm, a rare complication of central nervous system tuberculosis — A report and review of literature. Neurol India. 2017; 65(3): 626-628. https://doi.org/10.4103/neuroindia.NI_1280_16.

[41] Kheir AEM, Ibrahim SA, Hamed AA, Yousif BM, Hamid FA. Brain tuberculoma, an unusual cause of stroke in a child with trisomy 21: a case report. J Med Case Rep. 2017; 11(1): 114. https://doi.org/10.1186/s13256-017-1258-7.

[42] Jaiswal M, Gandhi A, Purohit D, Mittal RS. Concurrent multiple intracranial and intramedullary conus tuberculoma: A rare case report. Asian J Neurosurg. 2017; 12(2): 331-333. https://doi.org/10.4103/1793-5482.143461.

[43] Chandra SR, Advani S, Kumar R, Prasad C, Pai AR. Factors determining the clinical spectrum, course and response to treatment, and complications in seronegative patients with central nervous system tuberculosis. J Neurosci Rural Pract. 2017; 8(2): 241-248. https://doi.org/10.4103/jnrp.jnrp_466_16.

[44] Synmon B, Das M, Kayal AK, Goswami M, Sarma J, Basumatary L, Bhowmick S. Clinical and radiological spectrum of intracranial tuberculosis: ahospital based study in Northeast India. Indian J Tuberc. 2017; 64(2): 109-118. https://doi.org/10.1016/j.ijtb.2016.11.011. Epub 2016 Dec 16.

[45] Boulahri T, Taous A, Berri MA, Traibi I, Rouimi A. Multiple meningeal and cerebral involvement revealing multifocal tuberculosis in an immunocompetent patient. Pan Afr Med J. 2016; 25: 231. https://doi.org/10.11604/pamj.2016.25.231.11074. eCollection 2016.

[46] Chaudhary V, Bano S, Garga UC. Central nervous system tuberculosis: an imaging perspective. Can Assoc Radiol J. 2017; 68(2): 161-170. https://doi.org/10.1016/j.carj.2016.10.007. Epub 2017 Mar 7.

[47] Wang LN, Wang L, Liu LM, Song YM, Li Y, Liu H. Atypical spinal tuberculosis involved noncontiguous multiple segments: case series report with literature review. Medicine (Baltimore). 2017; 96(14): e6559. https://doi.org/10.1097/MD.0000000000006559.

[48] Pati S, De S, Ghosh TN, Ghosh MK. Multifocal pure tubercular osteomyelitis: an unusual presentation in childhood. Indian J Tuberc. 2017; 64(2): 136-140. https://doi.org/10.1016/j.ijtb.2016.01.004. Epub 2016 Jun 16.

[49] Leonard JM. Central nervous system tuberculosis. Microbiol Spectr. 2017; 5(2) https://doi.org/10.1128/microbiolspec.TNMI7-0044-2017.

[50] Gao Y, Ou Y, Deng Q, He B, Du X, Li J. Comparison between titanium mesh

and autogenous iliac bonegraft to restore vertebral height through posterior approach for the treatment of thoracic and lumbar spinal tuberculosis. PLoS One. 2017; 12(4): e0175567. https://doi.org/10.1371/journal.pone.0175567.eCollection 2017.

[51] Ye C, Hu X, Yu X, Zeng J, Dai M. Misdiagnosis of cystic tuberculosis of the olecranon. Orthopade. 2017; 46(5): 451-453. https://doi.org/10.1007/s00132-017-3401-y.

[52] Karakaplan M, Köroğlu M, Ergen E, Aslantürk O, Özdemir ZM, Ertem K. Isolated tuberculosis of capitate and triquetrum. J Wrist Surg. 2017; 6(1): 70-73. https://doi.org/10.1055/s-0036-1584312. Epub 2016 May 30.

[53] Grover SB, Arora S, Kumar A, Grover H, Katyan A, Nair DM. "Caught by the eye of sound" -epigastric swelling due to xiphisternal tuberculosis. Pol J Radiol. 2017; 82: 41-45. https://doi.org/10.12659/PJR.899329. eCollection 2017.

[54] Ayoub F, Khullar V, Powers H, Pham A, Islam S, Hematochezia SA. An uncommon presentation of colonic tuberculosis. Case Rep Gastrointest Med. 2017; 2017: 7831907. https://doi.org/10.1155/2017/7831907. Epub 2017 Apr 3.

[55] Singh SK, Srivastava A, Kumari N, Poddar U, Yachha SK, Pandey CM. Differentiation Between Crohn's Disease and Intestinal Tuberculosis in Children. J Pediatr Gastroenterol Nutr. 2018; 66(1): e6-e11. https://doi.org/10.1097/MPG.0000000000001625.

[56] Lakhe P, Khalife A, Pandya J. Ileocaecal and transverse colonic tuberculosis mimicking colonic malignancy — A case report. Int J Surg Case Rep. 2017; 36: 4-7. https://doi.org/10.1016/j.ijscr.2017.04.016. Epub ahead of print.

[57] Espinoza-Ríos J, Bravo Paredes E, Pinto Valdivia J, Guevara J, Huerta-Mercado J, Tagle Arróspide M, Bussalleu Rivera A. Penetrating gastric ulcer as a manifestation of multisystemic tuberculosis. Rev Gastroenterol Peru. 2017; 37(1): 91-93.

[58] Arai J, Kitamura K, Yamamiya A, Ishii Y, Nomoto T, Honma T, et al. Peripancreatic tuberculous lymphadenitis diagnosed via endoscopic ultrasound-guided fine-needle aspiration and polymerase chain reaction. Intern Med. 2017; 56(9): 1049-1052. https://doi.org/10.2169/internalmedicine.56.7509. Epub 2017 May 1.

[59] Marcianes P, Negro S, García-García L, Montejo C, Barcia E, Fernández-Carballido A. Surface-modified gatifloxacin nanoparticles with potential for treating central nervous system tuberculosis. Int J Nanomedicine. 2017; 12: 1959-1968. https://doi.org/10.2147/IJN.S130908. eCollection 2017.

2
结核性胸膜炎

内克拉·埃伦·图莱克

2.1 前言

结核病是世界上最致命的疾病之一。肺结核主要导致肺部组织病变，但它可能累及几乎全身所有的器官和组织。胸膜是由脏层胸膜和壁层胸膜两个部分组成，它包绕在肺组织周围，将肺脏与胸壁分隔开。结核性胸膜炎或结核性胸腔积液是成人肺外结核（EPTB）的第二种常见类型，仅次于淋巴受累。在结核病流行地区或发展中国家，结核性胸膜炎是胸腔积液的最常见原因，在发达国家，结核性胸膜炎导致的胸腔积液是继肿瘤、肺炎和心力衰竭之后的第四大原因[1,2]。从全球来看，肺结核发病率总体呈下降趋势，但由于HIV感染者和免疫功能低下患者的增加，EPTB的发病率却有所增加。结核性胸膜炎的原因主要有两种：一种是结核性胸膜炎病灶的原发感染，另一种则可能是由于先前存在的结核病灶继发感染所致。

2.2 流行病学

根据世界卫生组织统计的数据，结核病已成为全球第九大死亡原因。据统计，2016年结核病在HIV阴性人群中造成130万人死亡，在HIV阳性人群中造成的死亡人数高达37.4万人，新发的肺结核病例约有1 040万人[3]。HIV的感染和免疫抑制剂的使用增加了结核病的发病率[5,6]。高达30%的结核病患者患有结核性胸腔积液（tuberculous pleural effusion，TPE）[4]。当然，结核病患者中结核性胸膜炎的发病率在不同国家，不同人群中也具有一定的差异性，例如在布隆迪、南非、津巴布韦、乌干达和东南亚等结核病患病率较高的国家，结核性胸膜炎在患者中的占比较高，且多为年轻患者。在发展中国家,结核病是导致 TPE 的主要原因,胸腔积液的患者中高达 80% 患有胸膜结核[1,2]。在结核发病率较低的国家,结核性胸膜炎在老年人多见,主要是由于陈旧性结核病灶活动从而继发感染导致的[5,6]。

2.3 发病机制

以往的研究因为无法证明结核分枝杆菌来源于胸膜液,结核性 TPE 被认为是由于结核分枝杆菌引起的迟发型超敏反应导致的。近年来随着新的诊断方法的发展,提高了实验室检查的敏感性,改变了以往对结核性胸膜炎发病机理的认识。现有的研究认为,当病灶同时累及肺和胸膜时,TPE 可能受两种机制的影响。其主要的原因可能由于胸膜邻近组织或器官原发感染灶直接蔓延扩散至胸膜腔所致;其次,可能由于原发感染病灶通过血源性播散传播所致,而没有明显的胸膜实质受累。结核杆菌的特异性抗原如蛋白质多糖复合物、脂阿拉伯甘露聚糖等可进入胸膜腔,激活细胞免疫反应,引起机体的迟发型超敏反应。结核杆菌侵入机体后,中性粒细胞最先做出反应,然后是巨噬细胞。巨噬细胞吞噬分枝杆菌后,将抗原呈递给 T 淋巴细胞,随后 T 淋巴细胞被激活并通过分泌干扰素、白细胞介素-2 等细胞因子促进巨噬细胞的活化。活化的巨噬细胞又进一步产生肿瘤坏死因子,白细胞介素-1 等细胞因子进一步促进淋巴细胞的活化[7]。胸膜毛细血管通透性增加、细胞因子介导的炎症反应和壁层胸膜淋巴管阻塞都是导致胸腔积液的重要机制,血清蛋白进入和白细胞聚集,进而形成肉芽肿[8]。换句话说,TPE 是病理性免疫反应的结果。经过长时间的感染,随着陈旧性原发病灶的活动而进展[9]。

单纯的结核性 TPE 很少会进展为结核性脓胸,但当原发病灶存在空洞样病变时,大量的结核杆菌可通过破裂的空洞或支气管胸膜瘘进入胸腔,从而形成结核性脓胸,其特点是脓液中含有大量的结核杆菌和中性粒细胞。

2.4 临床表现

肺结核的临床表现因患者免疫功能、胸腔积液量及肺部受累部位的差异而有所不同,胸腔积液可以是少量的、中等的及大量的。通常,胸膜炎在初次感染结核杆菌后常有 3~6 个月的潜伏期,临床可无任何症状,可自行好转,但以后有复发的风险。胸膜受累多数是单侧的,约占90%左右,仅10%的患者双侧受累[9,10]。初次感染患者常呈急性或亚急性起病,临床表现主要为发热(85%)、干咳(75%)、胸痛(70%)、盗汗、乏力等,较少出现呼吸困难,发生大量胸腔积液时除外[11]。查体可见肺部听诊呼吸音减弱,叩诊呈浊音,当发生在疾病流行地区的年轻患者时,应注意与细菌性肺炎导致的TPE鉴别。

老年人和免疫功能低下的患者起病可能更为隐匿,当这类患者出低热、体重减轻、乏力和盗汗等临床表现时,应注意与充血性心力衰竭、肾衰、肺炎或肺栓塞等疾病相鉴别。其他的体征和症状,如盗汗、腹泻、淋巴结肿大和肝脾肿大等可在HIV感染的患者出现。如果出现胸膜纤维化和增厚加重,慢性胸痛和呼吸困难是最突出的症状,肺功能也会受到损害[9,11]。

2.5 诊断

如果患者有胸腔积液,且有与结核病相关的流行病学危险因素,如既往病史、结核病暴露史、家族史、曾居住或曾到过结核病流行地区,则应高度怀疑结核性TPE。痰液、胸膜液或胸膜活检标本中显示结核分枝杆菌阳性是诊断结核性TPE的主要依据。胸膜干酪样或上皮样细胞肉芽肿伴抗酸杆菌阳性的组织学表现也具有一定诊断价值。疑似TPE患者的初步评估应包括肺结核的诊断评估及影像学检查、痰中抗酸杆菌检查、结核培养和核酸扩增实验的结果[12],其外周血白细胞计数通常在正常范围。

结核性TPE的胸片常表现为单侧胸腔积液,多见于右半侧胸。仅在不到10%的病例发生双侧积液,其中约20%的TPE患者有同侧同时存在肺实质病变。结核性脓胸常伴有明显的肺实质病变,高分辨率胸部CT较胸部平片常具有更高的敏感性,在40%~85%的病例中,CT可以显示肺部微小结节、小叶间隔增厚等肺实质改变[13]。胸部超声可以准确定位积液位置,为穿刺抽液进行定位[14]。

即使在没有侵犯肺实质的情况下,痰抗酸杆菌涂片和结核分枝杆菌培养也可能呈阳性,其中HIV感染者的阳性结果较高[15,16]。

当TPE达到一定的量时,应进行诊断性胸穿抽液活检。取样后应分析TPE标本中的各类细胞计数、生化(蛋白质、葡萄糖、pH、乳酸脱氢酶等)和微生物(抗酸杆菌涂片培养、革兰染色培养、PCR等)情况,如果TPE以淋巴

2 结核性胸膜炎

细胞为主,应进一步分析样本的腺苷脱氨酶水平。正常 TPE 具有外观清澈、pH 在 7.60~7.64、白细胞<1 000/mm³、蛋白质含量<50%、蛋白质含量低于血清水平的 50%(1~2 g/dl)、乳酸脱氢酶低于血清水平的 50%、葡萄糖含量与血糖值相等特点。根据 Light 的标准,结核性 TPE 是一种淡黄色的渗出性液体,部分样本可带有一点点血色,pH<7.40,白细胞计数为 100~5 000/μl,淋巴细胞占 60%~90%,疾病早期可见多形核白细胞,嗜酸性粒细胞增多少见,当嗜酸性粒细胞超过 10%是则应考虑另外的诊断[17]。不典型的表现有脓性、乳糜和假性乳糜等,临床上比较少见,尤其是结核性脓胸[18]。结核性胸腔积液的蛋白含量应>3.0 g/dl,占血清蛋白浓度的 50%以上,并可检出>5 μg/dl 的高蛋白。葡萄糖水平可能正常,也可能降低。乳酸脱氢酶水平在大约 75%的病例中升高,即>500 U/L。

由于健康患者的胸膜内很少有微生物存在,因此抗酸涂片的敏感性非常低,阳性检出率低于<10%,但在 HIV 阳性的患者中,结核性 TPE 的患者由于其杆菌数量较高,其阳性率也有所增高,可达 20%左右[19,20]。所有原因不明的 TPE 患者都应进行诊断性穿刺抽液培养。在确诊为 TPE 的患者中,只有 20%~40%的患者通过抽液培养分离出结核分枝杆菌,但在 HIV 阳性患者中,培养阳性率稍高。痰培养与 TPE 培养相结合,可将结核分枝杆菌的检出率提高到 80%[21,22]。固体或液体培养基都可以使用,但液体培养基的敏感性更好,而且培养周期比固体培养基短[23]。虽然核酸扩增试验比传统方法更快,也可以直接检测临床标本中的结核分枝杆菌,但即使是使用 Xpert MTB/RIF 检测结核性胸膜炎导致的 TPE 仍存在低敏感性的问题,更好的检测方法仍有待进一步研究[24-27]。

通过组织学检查(上皮样细胞、干酪性和非干酪性肉芽肿)、抗酸染色和细针穿刺活检可确诊约 65%~75%的结核性胸膜炎患者[28]。此外,通过这些检查可以将结核性 TPE 与其他疾病如肿瘤、感染等引起的 TPE 很好地鉴别开来,与盲目活检相比,影像学检查引导下的活检和胸腔镜下的活检的诊断率更高[29,30]。

仅有 30%~40%的胸膜结核患者 PPD 试验呈阳性,但应注意在某些免疫抑制的患者常出现假阴性结果,PPD 阳性仅在结核低发区具有较高的诊断指导意义。同样,T-SPOT 阳性对于区分活动性结核和潜伏性感染无显著意义。这两种检查都不推荐用于结核性胸膜炎的诊断[31,32]。

目前的诊断检验方法既困难又费时,而且结果也不够理想。除此之外,样本的质量、检测方法和患者相关因素等都可能对实验结果产生影响。

因此,TPE生物标志物如腺苷脱氨酶、干扰素-γ、干扰素-γ诱导的10 kDa蛋白、白细胞介素-27、胸腔液溶菌酶浓度、新蝶呤、瘦素和其他的许多细胞因子,被期待能够用于简便快速的诊断结核性TPE。腺苷脱氨酶(adenosine deaminase,ADA)是嘌呤回收途径中的一种酶,其主要作用是催化腺苷和2-脱氧腺苷脱氨。结核分枝杆菌感染机体后,激活机体淋巴细胞发生体液免疫可以活化该酶,在疾病的早期即可被检测到。许多研究表明,胸膜ADA>40 U/L对以淋巴细胞为主的TPE的早期诊断具有较高的敏感性(92%)和特异性(90%),即使在抗酸涂片及杆菌培养阴性的患者,甚至在$CD4^+$ T细胞非常低的HIV阳性患者中也是如此[33,34]。ADA的低表达可用于结核低发地区排除性诊断[35]。由于胸膜间皮瘤、肿瘤、细菌性脓胸、类风湿性关节炎、淋巴瘤和肺炎导致的TPE等疾病ADA水平也会升高,反之高龄则可能降低,因此ADA的表达水平应与患者的临床表现和其他实验室结果共同作为诊断参考标准[36,37,38]。干扰素-γ是一种由活化的$CD4^+$ T细胞、细胞毒性T细胞和自然杀伤细胞释放的促炎细胞因子,可增强巨噬细胞吞噬分枝杆菌的活性。在结核性胸腔积液中检测到高水平的干扰素-γ,具有类似于ADA的高敏感性和特异性,但由于缺乏适宜的参考值范围从而使得其运用于临床诊断具有一定的局限性[39,40]。白细胞介素-27是由抗原提呈细胞分泌的一种细胞因子,介导干扰素-γ的产生和辅助性T细胞的活化,测定TPE中IL-27的水平可能有助于结核性胸膜炎的诊断,尤其是结合ADA的分泌情况[41,42]。当胸膜生物标志物水平与其他生物标志物和临床检验结果综合分析时,对结核性胸膜炎的诊断具有较大意义,但尚无特异性较强的生物标志物可直接诊断结核性胸膜炎,关于生物标志物在结核性胸膜炎病中的诊断还有待进一步研究[43,44]。

2.6 鉴别诊断

发生胸腔积液的原因多种多样,如恶性肿瘤(肺癌、乳腺癌)、充血性心力衰竭、肺炎(细菌、病毒、真菌)、脓肿(肝、膈下、脾)、炎性疾病(系统性红斑狼疮、类风湿性关节炎、丘格施特劳斯综合征、韦格纳肉芽肿)、肺栓塞、淋巴管异常等[2]。在发生不明原因的TPE时,诊断性胸膜腔穿刺取样进行标本分析可有助于明确诊断[45]。但仍有1/4的渗出性TPE患者未能通过TPE

活检明确诊断,可能还需要进一步进行胸膜活检。在肉芽肿性胸膜炎的鉴别诊断中必须考虑真菌感染、血管炎、自身免疫性疾病和结节病[46]。

2.7 治疗

大多数结核性胸腔积液可自行吸收,但复发的风险很高,在未经治疗的患者中,近2/3的患者在2～5年内发展为活动性肺结核或EPTB。由于未经治疗的结核性胸膜炎患者往往病程更长,同时更可能出现各种并发症,因此,所有结核性TPE患者均应进行治疗。在治疗前,应尽量对标本进行培养和药敏试验,至少应对异烟肼和利福平进行药敏试验。

其中,痰结核分枝杆菌阳性的患者应予以隔离,且所有结核性TPE的患者都应该进行HIV感染检测。

对临床上难以明确诊断的患者,可根据其临床表现、胸腔积液生化结果并排除其他可能的潜在病因,或胸膜活检显示肉芽肿性病变进行经验性抗结核治疗[1]。TPE的治疗方案与标准活动性肺结核相同,除了标准的抗结核化疗和胸腔引流外,皮质类固醇的使用对部分患者也具有一定的疗效。

结核性胸膜炎的治疗与肺结核一样,异烟肼＋利福平＋乙胺丁醇＋吡嗪酰胺＋吡哆醇治疗2个月,然后再用异烟肼＋利福平治疗4个月[47,48,49]。建议直接观察治疗和每日给药,不建议在整个治疗过程中每周给药3次。如果结核性胸膜炎是由多耐药结核杆菌引起的,应根据药敏结果选择合适的治疗方案,但对已经确诊的病例,尽管药敏试验结果报告未出,应先开始经验性治疗方案,然后根据检测结果调整治疗方案。如果治疗有效,症状常在2周内基本缓解,TPE则在6周内完全吸收,但部分患者发热和TPE的持续时间可能会分别延长至2个月和4个月。对于HIV阳性或生活在HIV高发区的患者和普通患者一样,应进行至少6个月的含有利福平的化疗方案,同时应考虑药物之间可能潜在的相互作用。

HIV感染患者开始化疗后的第一个月内很可能出现免疫重建炎症综合征(immune reconstitution inflammatory syndrome, IRIS),未感染HIV的患者也可能发生结核IRIS,尤其是胸膜和淋巴结受累长达3个月的患者,因此所有患者在治疗期间都必须密切随访,评估病情[50]。

皮质类固醇的联合用药可以缩短患者的病程和TPE的持续时间。对于有严重全身症状的患者,短期使用糖皮质激素可对病情有一定的缓解,还有助于减轻痊愈后胸膜增厚和胸膜粘连的程度,但对肺功能的长远影响尚不清楚[51]。由于会增加机会性感染和患卡波西肉瘤的风险,所以对 HIV 阳性的患者使用激素目前还较为谨慎[52]。

对于结核性 TPE 的患者,不推荐常规引流 TPE,如果患者有大量 TPE 导致呼吸困难时,可考虑进行治疗性胸膜腔穿刺以缓解症状,结核性脓胸患者可能需要切开引流[53]。

胸膜增厚、纤维化、慢性胸痛、肺功能受损和呼吸困难是结核性 TPE 常见的并发症。抗结核治疗结束后发生胸膜增厚概率在 5%~55%,但多数随着病程的延长而降低。虽然有一些数据表明纤溶剂的使用对后遗症胸膜增厚的发生具有一定的疗效,但数据还不够充分,仍需要进一步研究。

参考文献

[1] Zhai K, Lu Y, Shi H-Z. Tuberculous pleural effusion. J Thoracic Dis. 2016; 8(7): E486-494. https://doi.org/10.21037/jtd.2016.05.87.

[2] Porcel JM, Esquerda A, Vives M, et al. Etiology of pleural effusions: analysis of more than 3000 consecutive thoracenteses. Arch Broncopneumol. 2014; 50: 161-165.

[3] Global tuberculosis report 2017. Geneva: World Health Organization; 2017 http://www.who.int/tb/publications/global_report/MainText_13Nov2017.pdf?ua=1. Accessed 25 Nov 2017.

[4] Qiu L, Teeter LD, Liu Z, Ma X, Musser JM, Ea G. Diagnostic associations between pleural and pulmonary tuberculosis. J Inf Secur. 2006; 53(6): 377-386.

[5] Golden MP, Vikram HR. Extrapulmonary tuberculosis: an overview. Am Fam Physician. 2005; 72(9): 1761-1768.

[6] Chamie G, Luetkemeyer A, Walusimbi-Nantenza M, et al. Significant variation in presentation of pulmonary tuberculosis across a high resolution of CD4 strata. Int J Tuberc Lung Dis. 2010; 14: 1295-1302.

[7] Cooper AM. Cell-mediated immune responses in tuberculosis. Annu Rev Immunol. 2009; 27(1): 393-422.

[8] Vorster MJ, Allwood BW, Diacon AH, Koegelenberg CFN. Tuberculous pleural effusions: advances and controversies. J Thoracic Dis. 2015; 7(6): 981-991.

[9] Porcel JM. Tuberculous pleural effusion. Lung. 2009; 187(5): 263-270.

[10] Jeong YJ, Lee KS. Pulmonary tuberculosis: up-to-date imaging and management. Am J Roentgenol. 2008; 191: 834-844.

[11] Porcel JM. Advances in the diagnosis of tuberculous pleuritis. Ann Transl Med. 2016; 4(15): 282. https://doi.org/10.21037/atm.2016.07.23.

[12] Mcgrath EE, Anderson PB. Diagnostic tests for tuberculous pleural effusion. Eur J Clin Microbiol Infect Dis. 2010; 29(10): 1187-1193.

[13] Seiscento M, Vargas FS, Bombarda S, et al. Pulmonary involvement in pleural

tuberculosis: how often does it mean disease activity. Respiratory Med. 2011; 105: 1079-1083.
[14] Koegelenberg CF, von Groote-Bidlingmaier F, Bolliger CT. Transthoracic ultrasonography for the respiratory physician. Respiration. 2012; 84: 337-350.
[15] Conde MB, Loivos AC, Rezende VM, et al. Yield of sputum induction in the diagnosis of pleural tuberculosis. Am J Respir Crit Care Med. 2003; 167: 723-725.
[16] Aljohaney A, Amjadi K, Alvarez GG. A systematic review of the epidemiology, immunopathogenesis, diagnosis, and treatment of pleural TB in HIV-infected patients. Clin Dev Immunol. 2012; 2012: 842045. https://doi.org/10.1155/2012/842045.
[17] Light RW, Macgregor MI, Luchsinger PC, Ball WC Jr. Pleural effusions: the diagnostic separation of transudates and exudates. Ann Intern Med. 1972; 77(4): 507-513.
[18] Jolobe OM. Atypical tuberculous pleural effusions. Eur J Inter Med. 2011; 22: 456-459.
[19] Kitinya JN, Richter C, Perenboom R, et al. Influence of HIV status on pathological changes in tuberculous pleuritis. Tuber Lung Dis. 1994; 75: 195-198.
[20] Marjani M, Yousefzadeh A, Baghaei P, et al. Impact of HIV infection on tuberculous pleural effusion. Int J STD AIDS. 2016; 27: 363-369.
[21] Ruan SY, Chuang YC, Wang JY, et al. Revisiting tuberculous pleurisy: pleural fluid characteristics and diagnostic yield of mycobacterial culture in an endemic area. Thorax. 2012; 67: 822-827.
[22] Ko Y, Song J, Lee SY, et al. Does repeated pleural culture increase the diagnostic yield of *Mycobacterium tuberculosis* from tuberculous pleural effusion in HIV-negative individuals? PLoS One. 2017; 12(7): e0181798. https://doi.org/10.1371/journal.pone.0181798.
[23] Rageade F, Picot N, Blanc-Michaud A, et al. Performance of solid and liquid culture media for the detection of Mycobacterium tuberculosis in clinical materials: metaanalysis of recent studies. Eur J Clin Microbiol Infect Dis. 2014; 33: 867-870.
[24] Denkinger CM, Schumacher SG, Boehme CC, et al. Xpert MTB/RIF assay for the diagnosis of extrapulmonary tuberculosis: a systematic review and meta-analysis. Eur Respir J. 2014; 44: 435-446.
[25] Saeed M, Ahmad M, Iram S, Riaz S, Akhtar M, Aslam M. GeneXpert technology A breakthrough for the diagnosis of tuberculous pericarditis and pleuritic in less than 2 hours. Saudi Med J. 2017; 38(7): 699-705.
[26] Trajman A, da Silva Santos Kleiz de Oliveira EF, Bastos ML, et al. Accuracy of polimerase chain reaction for the diagnosis of pleural tuberculosis. Respir Med. 2014; 108: 918-923.
[27] Sehgal IS, Dhooria S, Aggarwal AN, et al. Diagnostic performance of xpert MTB/RIF in tuberculous pleural effusion: systematic review and meta-analysis. J Clin Microbiol. 2016; 54: 1133-1136.
[28] Sahn SA, Huggins JT, San José ME, et al. Can tuberculous pleural effusions be diagnosed by pleural fluid analysis alone? Int J Tuberc Lung Dis. 2013; 17: 787-793.

[29] DePew ZS, Maldonado F. The role of interventional therapy for pleural diseases. Expert Rev Respir Med. 2014; 8(4): 465-477.

[30] Bibby AC, Maskell NA. Pleural biopsies in undiagnosed pleural effusions: Abrams vs image-guided vs thoracoscopic biopsies. Curr Opin Pulm Med. 2016; 22(4): 392-398.

[31] Gopi A, Madhavan SM, Sharma SK, et al. Diagnosis and treatment of tuberculous pleural effusion in 2006. Chest. 2007; 131: 880-889.

[32] Aggarwal AN, Agarwal R, Gupta D, Dhooria S, Behera D. Interferon gamma release assays for diagnosis of pleural tuberculosis: a systematic review and meta-analysis. Carroll KC, ed. J Clin Microbiol. 2015; 53(8): 2451-2459.

[33] Villegas MV, Labrada LA, Saravia NG. Evaluation of polymerase chain reaction, adenosine deaminase, and interferon-gamma in pleural fluid for the differential diagnosis of pleural tuberculosis. Chest. 2000; 118: 1355-1364.

[34] Baba K, Hoosen AA, Langeland N, Dyrhol-Riise AM. Adenosine deaminase activity is a sensitive marker for the diagnosis of tuberculous pleuritis in patients with very low CD4 counts. Zaas AK, ed. PLoS One. 2008; 3(7): e2788. https://doi.org/10.1371/journal.pone.0002788.

[35] Arnold DT, Bhatnagar R, Fairbanks LD, et al. Pleural Fluid Adenosine Deaminase (Pfada) in the diagnosis of tuberculous effusions in a low incidence population. Caylà JA, ed. PLoS ONE. 2015; 10(2): e0113047. https://doi.org/10.1371/journal.pone.0113047.

[36] Liang QL, Shi HZ, Wang K, Qin SM, Qin XJ. Diagnostic accuracy of adenosine deaminase in tuberculous pleurisy: a meta-analysis. Respir Med. 2008; 102(5): 744-754.

[37] Jiménez Castro D, Díaz Nuevo G, Pérez-Rodríguez E, Light RW. Diagnostic value of adenosine deaminase in nontuberculous lymphocytic pleural effusions. Eur Respir J. 2003; 21(2): 220-224.

[38] Light RW. Update on tuberculous pleural effusion. Respirology. 2010; 15: 451-458.

[39] Wang H, Yue J, Yang J, Gao R, Liu J. Clinical diagnostic utility of adenosine deaminase, interferon-γ, interferon-γ-induced protein of 10 kDa, and dipeptidyl peptidase 4 levels in tuberculous pleural effusions. Heart Lung. 2012; 41(1): 70-75. https://doi.org/10.1016/j.hrtlng.2011.04.049.

[40] Jiang J, Shi HZ, Liang QL, Qin SM, Qin XJ. Diagnostic value of interferon-γ in tuberculous pleurisy: a meta-analysis. Chest. 2007; 2007131(4): 1133-1141.

[41] Wu YB, Ye ZJ, Qin SM, Wu C, Chen YQ, Shi HZ. Combined detections of interleukin 27, interferon-γ, and adenosine deaminase in pleural effusion for diagnosis of tuberculous pleurisy. Chin Med J (Engl). 2013; 126(17): 3215-3221.

[42] Skouras VS, Magkouta SF, Psallidas I, et al. Interleukin-27 improves the ability of adenosine deaminase to rule out tuberculous pleural effusion regardless of pleural tuberculosis prevalence. Infect Dis (Lond). 2015; 47: 477-483.

[43] Wallis RS, Kim P, Cole S, et al. Tuberculosis biomarkers discovery: developments, needs, and challenges. Lancet Infect Dis. 2013; 13(4): 362-372.

[44] Zeng N, Wan C, Qin J, et al. Diagnostic value of interleukins for tuberculous pleural effusion: a systematic review and meta-analysis. BMC Pulm Med. 2017;

17: 180. https://doi.org/10.1186/s12890-017-0530-3.
[45] Porcel JM, Azzopardi M, Koegelenberg CF, et al. The diagnosis of pleural effusions. Expert Rev Respir Med. 2016; 9: 801-815.
[46] Maldonado F, Lentz RJ, Light RW. Diagnostic approach to pleural diseases: new tricks for an old trade. F1000Res. 2017; 17(6): 1135. https://doi.org/10.12688/f1000research.11646.1.
[47] Guidelines for treatment of drug-susceptible tuberculosis and patient care (2017 update). Geneva: World Health Organization; 2017. Licence: CC BY-NC-SA 3.0 IGO.
[48] Nahid P, Dorman SE, Alipanah N, et al. Official American Thoracic Society/Centers for Disease Control and Prevention/Infectious Diseases Society of America Clinical Practice Guidelines. Treatment of drug-susceptible tuberculosis. Clin Infect Dis. 2016; 63(7): e147-95. https://doi.org/10.1093/cid/ciw376.
[49] Dheda K, Barry CE, Maartens G. Tuberculosis. Lancet. 2016; 387: 1211-1226.
[50] Geri G, Passeron A, Heym B, et al. Paradoxical reactions during treatment of tuberculosis with extrapulmonary manifestations in HIV-negative patients. Infection. 2013; 41(2): 537-543.
[51] Ryan H, Yoo J, Darsini P. Corticosteroids for tuberculous pleurisy. Cochrane Database Syst Rev. 2017; (3): CD001876. https://doi.org/10.1002/14651858.CD001876.pub3.
[52] Elliott AM, Luzze H, Quigley MA, et al. A randomized, double-blind, placebo-controlled trial of the use of prednisolone as an adjunct to treatment in HIV-1-associated pleural tuberculosis. J Infect Dis. 2004; 190: 869-878.
[53] Bhuniya S, Arunabha DC, Choudhury S, et al. Role of therapeutic thoracentesis in tuberculous pleural effusion. Ann Thorac Med. 2012; 7: 215-219.

3
胃肠结核和结核性腹膜炎

索菲娅·德·萨拉姆和乔恩·S. 弗里德兰

3.1 流行病学

在抗生素出现之前,肺结核患者尸检显示高达90%的病例有肠道受累[30]。在当前时期,获取有关胃肠结核(gastrointestinal tuberculosis, GI TB)的准确数据受到一些因素的限制。在许多资源匮乏的情况下,传染性肺部疾病的诊断、治疗和报告要优先于肺外疾病。在某些情况下,由于获得诊断的途径有限,无法确认胃肠结核。在许多情况下,报告系统的准确性是可变的。队列研究虽然对收集详细信息有用,但往往会受到选择偏差的影响,例如,外科中心报告的队列可能会夸大需要手术的胃肠结核患者比率。

考虑到这些限制,现有的数据表明,GI TB的流行病学在世界各地差异很大。在欧洲和美国,它是第六位最常见的肺外结核(EPTB)好发部位[65,74],而在沙特阿拉伯,GI TB是EPTB最常见的部位[1]。在英国,印度次大陆患者的腹部结核发病率是白人患者的3倍[71]。GI TB好发于年轻人,平均年龄在30岁末到40岁初[8,36]。在尼日利亚,10%的腹部结核诊断病例为儿童[36],而在欧洲,儿童仅占诊断病例的3.7%[74]。性别分布各不相同,印度和巴基斯坦以女性居多[10,18],而沙特阿拉伯和英国的性别分布则相同[1,8]。

虽然大多数培养确诊的GI TB病例是由结核分枝杆菌引起的[55],但由牛分枝杆菌引起的人畜共患结核病在某些情况下仍占相当大的比率,而且很可能全世界牛分枝杆菌的影响没有得到充分报道。牛分枝杆菌引起的结核病(在所有解剖部位中)的比率显示出很大的地域差异,非洲占2.8%,美洲占0.3%,欧洲占0.4%,来自亚洲和西太平洋的数据非常少[59]。在美国加利福尼亚州的一个队列中,牛分枝杆菌占成人结核病诊断的8%,占儿童结核病诊断的一半[72]。在加利福尼亚州的队列中,97%的诊断为西班牙裔。在英国感染牛分枝杆菌的人群中有 3/4 出生在英国,而在英国引入广泛的牛奶消毒技术之前,也有类似比率的婴儿出生[53]。牛结核杆菌流行病学的变化可能与对牛结核病控制水平的变化、食用未经巴氏杀菌的乳制品的模式和迁移有关。

特定人群罹患胃肠结核的风险较高。HIV 感染者患各种 EPTB 的风险更高,在一些合并感染的人群中,GI TB 已被报告为肺外最常见的部位[37]。在资源丰富的环境中,HIV 感染患者牛分枝杆菌发病率的相对危险度是 HIV 阴性患者 2.6~8.3 倍[59]。该相关危险度尚未在资源匮乏的环境中证实。

接受抗 TNF-α 治疗的患者感染结核病的风险增加。包括 GI TB 在内的肺外疾病的比率高于肺结核现有的比率[41]。结核性腹膜炎尽管很少发生在接受持续不卧床腹膜透析(continuous ambulatory peritoneal dialysis,CAPD)的患者中。报告的病例中有 69% 没有腹膜外疾病,也没有确定的结核病危险因素[82]。体外研究表明,pH 和渗透压的改变可能会损害腹腔液中白细胞的功能[42],我们实验室正在进行的研究表明,酸中毒可以调节许多结核特异性免疫反应。因此,CAPD 可能会增加结核性腹膜炎的风险。

在资源丰富的环境中,酒精性肝病(alcoholic liver disease,ALD)与结核性腹膜炎风险增加有关。在一项研究中,62% 的结核性腹膜炎患者患有 ALD[76]。这种关联的强度在资源贫乏环境下的队列中看不到。这种联系的原因尚不完全清楚,但可能与 ALD 相关的营养不良及随后的 T 细胞损伤有关。

3.2 发病机制

GI TB 的主要病原体(结核分枝杆菌)可通过以下途径感染消化道：吞咽从肺部病灶排出的含结核分枝杆菌的痰液;从身体其他部位的活动性结核病灶经淋巴或血源性传播;从邻近器官直接传播或摄入受污染的乳制品。

由牛分枝杆菌引起的 GI TB 主要通过摄入未经巴氏灭菌的牛奶和奶制品传播,但也可以通过吸入空气中的牛分枝杆菌从动物传染给人类,极少数情况下也会从人传染给人。

当结核分枝杆菌从痰液或受污染的食品中被摄取时,在吞噬杆菌的 M 细胞帮助下进入肠道黏膜。M 细胞将杆菌呈递给黏膜相关淋巴组织的滤泡旁区域的树突状细胞和巨噬细胞。组织内的分枝杆菌和巨噬细胞以及单核细胞来源的未成熟巨噬细胞内的分枝杆菌能够逃脱杀死,并进行细胞内的循环复制,释放到细胞外空间。一些被感染的巨噬细胞可能通过淋巴或血源性途径传播。在γ-干扰素和肿瘤坏死因子α的支持下,T淋巴细胞与成熟巨噬细胞的相互作用导致肉芽肿的形成。破坏维持这些肉芽肿的平衡会导致肉芽肿液化、基质金属蛋白酶辅助的组织损伤和分枝杆菌的释放[24,32,49,70]。对结核病免疫病理的详细回顾超出了本章的范围,但尚未对胃肠道特异因素进行任何详细的研究或定义。

GI TB好发于回盲部,这是由于肠内淋巴组织丰富,以及肠内容物与肠黏膜接触时间相对较长所致。青壮年肠道相关淋巴组织密度较高也可能部分解释了该年龄段GI TB发病率较高的原因[23]。

3.3 临床表现

结核病的临床表现与其他疾病非常类似,这一点对于GI TB来说尤其如此。GI TB的临床表现可能是非特异性的,并根据疾病的具体部位和宿主的免疫状态而变化。它与炎症性肠病、胃肠道感染(如阿米巴病、肠热病和小肠结肠炎耶尔森氏菌)以及胃肠道或其他腹腔和盆腔器官恶性肿瘤的临床表现相似。只有15%～25%的GI TB患者同时患有活动性肺结核[35,55]。这些因素往往导致GI TB诊断的延迟,并导致发病率和死亡率的增加。GI TB的诊断需要提高怀疑指数。

3.3.1 肠道结核

虽然大多数肠结核患者都有潜在的症状,平均症状持续时间为5～8个月,但据报道,大约1/3的患者出现了急腹症[1,45,64]。肠结核患者最常见的症状是腹痛(40%～100%)、体重减轻(30%～80%)、发热(30%～60%)、恶心和呕吐(15%～50%)和排便习惯改变(高达50%)[1,27,29,45,64,71]。肠道内疾病的确切位置决定了主要的表现特征。至少一半的肠结核患者在胃肠道的多个位置都有病变。

3.3.1.1 食管结核

食管病变仅占所有GI TB的0.2%～1%[1,29,35,71]。最常见的症状是吞咽困难,但可能包括伴随症状有食欲缺乏,体重减轻,胸骨后疼痛,很少见出血。与呼吸道或纵隔淋巴结结核相关的气管食管瘘和纵隔食管瘘的形成已被描述[38,66]。

3.3.1.2 胃结核

高达2%的肠结核病变位于胃内。主要症状包括腹痛、恶心、呕吐和体重减轻。临床和内镜特征与消化性溃疡或胃恶性肿瘤相似。表现为幽门梗阻的胃结核也已被描述[19,29]。

3.3.1.3 小肠结核

1/3~1/2的肠结核患者有小肠受累[1,29]。腹痛、恶心呕吐、腹胀和发热是最常见的主诉。在以急腹症表现的胃肠结核的队列中，小肠狭窄占1/2[10]。

3.3.1.4 回盲肠结核

回盲部是肠结核最常见的部位，高达80%的肠结核患者累及此部位[27,44,64,71]。最常见的主诉是腹痛，可能是全腹广泛性的或位于右侧髂窝。1/2的患者还会出现呕吐、体重减轻和腹泻。在25%~50%的患者中，右下腹可触摸到腹部肿块[35]，可能被误认为恶性肿块或阑尾脓肿。

3.3.1.5 结肠结核

大约10%的肠结核患者有结肠病变。最常见的症状是体重减轻、腹痛、发热、食欲缺乏和排便习惯的改变。据报道，1/3的患者出现血性腹泻，可类似痢疾[29]。阑尾受影响的比率为2%~3%[29,45]，表现方式与急性阑尾炎或阑尾脓肿相似。多达1/2的结肠或阑尾受累患者可触及腹部肿块。

3.3.1.6 肛门直肠结核

肛门直肠受累很少见，仅发生在1%的肠结核病例中。它可表现为直肠肿块或肛门直肠瘘[1,29]。

3.3.2 肠结核与克罗恩病的鉴别

克罗恩病与胃肠结核的鉴别诊断最复杂，特别是在较发达的国家，因为临床和内镜特征非常相似，而且这两种疾病都好发于回盲部。有证据表明，克罗恩病在一些发展中国家的发病率正在增加，在一个队列中，43%最终被诊断为克罗恩病的患者以前曾接受过抗结核治疗[17]。

临床特征可有助于鉴别这两种疾病的存在,肛周疾病在克罗恩病中更常见,以及高热,如果没有腹腔脓肿,则提示是 GI TB。增大、坏死的淋巴结和腹水或腹膜增厚在计算机断层扫描中已在 GI TB 中被描述,但在克罗恩病中未见描述[13]。内镜特征不能可靠的区分这两种疾病,但纵向溃疡、肛门直肠受累和鹅卵石外观在克罗恩病中更为常见,而横向溃疡和扩张的回盲瓣提示 GI TB 常见[28,46]。正如下面所讨论的,微生物学诊断价值不高,意味着组织学是鉴别这两种疾病的关键方式。组织学检查中出现融合性或坏死性肉芽肿高度提示 GI TB,干酪样坏死本质上可诊断[2]。最近发表的一个模型显示,在小型验证队列中识别 GI TB 的灵敏度和特异度超过 90%[47]。这需要在更大的多国队列中进一步验证。

3.3.3 结核性腹膜炎

结核性腹膜炎的主要临床特征是腹水(73%)、腹痛(65%)(通常是非局限性的)、体重减轻(61%)、发热(59%)和腹部压痛(48%)[73]。一小部分(5%~10%)有干性或粘连性结核性腹膜炎,并伴有少量腹水。5%的患者出现继发性粘连性小肠梗阻[15]。腹膜结核的临床影像、腹水和腹腔镜特征很难与腹膜癌相鉴别。

3.3.4 HIV 感染患者的表现

HIV 阳性患者感染 GI TB 的临床表现在某些方面与 HIV 阴性患者感染 GI TB 不同。在 HIV 阳性者中,GI TB 与播散性结核相关的可能性高出 HIV 阴性者 3 倍。高热、盗汗和体重减轻的临床症状明显比 HIV 阴性的人更常见。在 HIV 感染的患者中,腹水是一个不太明显的特征,而腹部淋巴结病变和脾及肝受累则更为常见[25]。与 HIV 相关的结核病只有在治疗逆转录病毒后和发展免疫重建炎症综合征(IRIS)后才会在临床上显现出来。

3.3.5 儿童中的表现

在儿童中,腹部结核影响腹膜、淋巴结和肠道本身的比率分别为 45%、

35％和20％。在多达25％的病例中,除腹膜或肠以外,还有淋巴结受累。通常表现为食欲缺乏、体重减轻(高达70％)和腹胀(50％)。多达50％患有GI TB的儿童出现在外科,10％的儿童在就诊时被发现有临床腹膜炎。与成人队列形成对比的是,一些儿科队列描述了多达50％～75％的儿童伴有胸部异常,其中高达40％的儿童出现胃肠外症状[22,57,83]。

3.4 调查研究

微生物学确诊胃肠结核的病例在10％～70％,具体取决于疾病的确切部位以及采样和诊断方式的可用性。在30％～40％的病例中,特征性组织学是主要的诊断手段。其余的诊断是根据临床、流行病学、放射学和组织学特征以及抗结核治疗的反应做出的。腹部淋巴结或远处解剖部位的样本的培养或组织学也可以提供支持证据[1,29,44,45,67,71]。

3.4.1 血液参数

GI TB患者血常规显示非特异性异常,贫血占60％,红细胞沉降率＞30 mm/h占67％,白细胞计数增高占28％[1,27,29,45]。

3.4.2 放射学

3.4.2.1 普通X线片和钡检查

高达25％～45％的患者胸部X线片检查异常,虽然大多数病例的改变是非特异性的,但这可能会增加结核病的怀疑指数[1,7,71,78]。在出现急腹症的患者中,直立胸片有助于寻找腹腔游离气体。腹部平片可显示钙化的淋巴结,在有狭窄或肠梗阻的患者中,可见扩张的肠袢。

钡剂检查显示50％～80％的肠道结核患者有异常。这些异常包括溃疡、狭窄、盲肠和回盲瓣畸形以及钡剂快速排空[18,27,35,44,52,57,71]。

3.4.2.2 超声

超声(ultrasound, US)对检测腹水很有用,特别是在腹水体积小但临床无法检测到的腹膜结核中。腹水也出现在1/3的肠道结核病例中,它的检测有助于区分肠结核和克罗恩病,因为后者很少出现腹水[2]。腹水内存在间隔、纤维蛋白束或碎片,虽然不是病原学依据,但增加了结核病的可能性。US 显示 25%～60%的病例有淋巴结病变,还显示肠系膜或肠壁增厚[43,44,57,73]。US 的一个主要局限性是,肠管及其相关的肠系膜或淋巴结的图像可能会被充气肠袢所遮挡覆盖。

3.4.2.3 计算机断层扫描

与超声相比,计算机断层扫描(computed tomography,CT)可以进一步表现出腹膜和淋巴结的变化特征,以及成像整个肠道。腹部 CT 静脉造影显示,40%～70%GI TB 患者中有增大的、周围增强的中央低密度淋巴结,呈干酪样坏死。其他与 GI TB 相关的淋巴结类型包括混合密度的淋巴结肿块,伴有肠袢或肠系膜的多发轻度增大的淋巴结和钙化的淋巴结。虽然淋巴结坏死或钙化不是结核病的特异性,但它们具有很高的提示性[81]。结核性的腹膜增厚在 CT 上的表现通常是光滑且明显强化,与癌性疾病的结节状、不规则增厚形成对比[33]。CT 上可能显示的其他异常包括肠壁增厚、狭窄、瘘管、炎性肿块和粘连(图 3-1)。

3.4.2.4 磁共振成像

在许多 GI TB 发病率最高的地区,磁共振成像(magnetic resonance imaging,MRI)并没有得到广泛应用。即使有,它也是一项更耗时、更昂贵的调查,因此,它通常只在特定情况下使用。例如,MRI 可以用来避免年轻

图 3-1 轴位增强 CT 图像显示小肠增厚、狭窄区域(中箭头),周围有肠系膜粘连。近端可见扩张小肠(上箭头),远端可见小肠塌陷(下箭头)。(感谢英国伦敦帝国理工学院医疗保健 NHS 信托基金会的艾莉森·格雷厄姆医生提供图片)

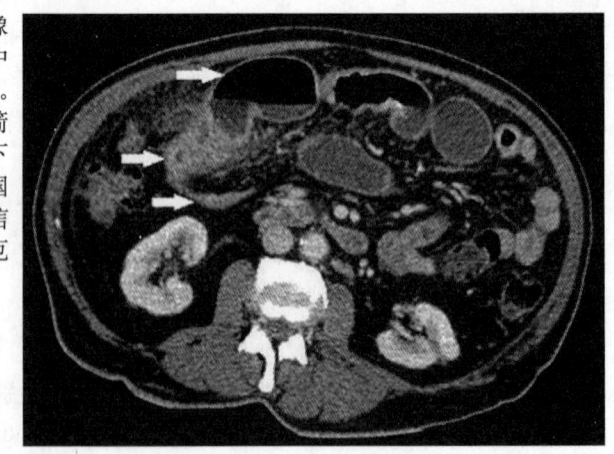

患者重复CT扫描的辐射暴露。在静脉造影剂不能使用或CT禁忌使用的情况下，MRI平扫比CT平扫能提供更多的信息。大多数MRI和CT的表现都不是GI TB的特异性表现，但分隔性和周围腹部淋巴结增强提示结核。MRI对淋巴结内钙化的检测灵敏度低于CT[39,77]。

3.4.2.5 功能成像

18F-脱氧葡萄糖正电子发射断层扫描/计算机断层扫描（18F-FDG PET/CT）使用放射性标记葡萄糖摄取来评估代谢活性。一项研究检查了其在鉴别腹膜增厚原因中的应用，发现这种方法不能可靠的区分恶性和结核性腹膜增厚，因为这两种疾病过程都与组织中葡萄糖摄取增加有关[14]。据我们所知，虽然有许多病例报告表明功能显像可能有一定作用，但目前还没有专门研究功能显像在肠道结核病中的应用。由于最常见的鉴别诊断，即炎症性肠病和恶性肿瘤，都可能导致葡萄糖摄取增加，因此功能成像似乎不太可能排除对组织取样的需要。

3.4.3 组织取样方法

3.4.3.1 经皮穿刺取样

如果有腹水，是最容易得到的标本。然而，如下所述，培养阳性率较低。盲法腹膜活检已经使用了几十年，由此产生的样本可以从组织学上确认40%～60%的患者腹膜结核的诊断。有记录的手术并发症包括肠穿孔和出血(1%～2%)及相关死亡率[11,75,80]。据报道，在成人和儿童队列中，放射引导下腹膜或腹腔淋巴结取样的阳性率都在50%左右[44,52]。在资源允许的情况下，直接可视化腹膜活检可提供更高的阳性率，如下所述。

3.4.3.2 内镜检查

肠结核在内镜下的肉眼特征包括溃疡、狭窄、结节、假性息肉和回盲部变形。当出现多个溃疡时，可穿插有不同长度的正常黏膜，如克罗恩病所见[84]。更多关于肠结核和克罗恩病的区别，见第3.3.2节。

在75%的病例中，内镜下病变活检可获得支持的组织学信息[27,44]。当黏膜异常超出常规内窥镜检查范围时，推进式内窥镜或逆行回肠镜检查可有用。视频胶囊内镜检查可在通过这些技术确定后续活检的靶点或本身记录小肠疾病的程度方面发挥作用[61,68]。内镜超声可用于评估和采样与食管病变相关的纵隔淋巴结[50,69]。

3.4.3.3 诊断性手术操作

通过手术直接观察病理来收集标本,可以提高组织学的诊断率。腹腔镜被广泛用于不明原因的腹水或腹膜增厚的检查。在结核性腹膜炎病例中,手术时最常见的肉眼表现是腹水、腹膜上的黄色或白色结节以及腹膜或内脏粘连。据报道,仅凭视觉表现的敏感度为84%~100%,特异度为96%~100%。手术活检标本组织学检查的敏感性为70%~100%,特异性接近100%。在较老的病例中,腹腔镜的并发症发生率为1.5%~3%[16,73],但现在几乎可以肯定,这一比率已经降低,特别是在由有经验的手术人员进行操作的情况下。

在无法进行腹腔镜检查的中心或有广泛腹膜粘连的情况下,剖腹手术可用于获取组织样本。在一些老年患者组中,50%的剖腹手术纯粹是为了诊断[57]。局部麻醉下腹膜切开活检是一种替代方法,已被一些中心使用[79]。

诊断性腹腔镜或开腹手术在肠结核中的作用是有限的。在现有的内镜方法无法触及肠道病变的情况下,外科方法允许对相关的肠系膜淋巴结进行采样[2]。

3.4.4 腹水分析

结核性腹膜炎患者的腹水标本中通常含有500~1 500个白细胞/mm^3,主要是淋巴细胞。然而,低白细胞计数并不排除结核性腹膜炎的可能,也可以发现以中性粒细胞为主,尤其是在肾衰竭患者中。直到目前,中性粒细胞在免疫病理学中的重要性也一直被忽视[63]。无肝硬化的几乎所有结核性腹膜炎患者的血清-腹水白蛋白梯度均小于11 g/L。然而,在伴有门脉高压腹水的患者中,敏感性及特异性均较低。当腹水腺苷脱氨酶水平≥30 U/L时,敏感性和特异性均≥90%。腹水中LDH、CA-125或葡萄糖的水平没有足够的鉴别性,不推荐常规检测[73]。

3.4.5 组织学和细胞学

在缺乏阳性微生物学的情况下,典型的组织学有助于高达75%的肠结核的诊断[44,71]。

3.4.5.1 肠结核

黏膜标本中的融合性肉芽肿和干酪性肉芽肿被认为是肠结核的诊断，但只有25%～50%的标本出现。60%～70%的样本中存在非干酪性肉芽肿，慢性炎症和溃疡是常见的表现，但并非肠结核特有的[2,28,44]。

在高达5%的肠结核病例中，肠组织的组织学表现为非特异性异常，而肉芽肿仅出现在相关的肠系膜淋巴结中。可能需要检查多个淋巴结以确定肉芽肿。

3.4.5.2 结核性腹膜炎

在直接目视下取样，70%～90%的标本为非干酪性肉芽肿，33%～100%的标本为干酪性肉芽肿。抗酸染色显示25%～75%的标本中有抗酸杆菌，即使腹膜的肉眼外观仅显示轻度红斑也可能呈抗酸染色阳性[34,54,60,76]。

3.4.6 微生物学

3.4.6.1 培养

结核性腹膜炎患者腹水抗酸染色阳性率仅为3%～6%，培养阳性率为16%～35%[60,73]。如果大量离心腹水，培养细胞颗粒，培养率可提高到66%～83%。腹膜组织阳性率较高，染色阳性率为50%，培养阳性率为70%以上。肠道组织标本培养阳性率为25%～35%[2,4,34,52]。金胺染色也更为敏感。

液体培养基的使用将检测分枝杆菌的时间从传统固体培养基的4~8周减少到了平均14天。使用液体培养基的另一个好处是，与标准的Lowenstein-Jensen培养基相比，它可以更好地支持牛分枝杆菌的生长[31]。廉价的快速检测，如显微镜观察药敏试验（microscopic observation drug susceptibility，MODS）[58]，可能对上消化道结核有效[48]。

3.4.6.2 核酸扩增技术

结核聚合酶链反应（polymerase chain reaction，PCR）提供了一种快速

诊断方法，但受到所需设备和实验室人员的限制。几项研究报告，针对 IS6100 基因区域的 PCR 对肠道组织样本的敏感性为 60%～65%，但对腹水样本的敏感性仅为 7%。PCR 的特异性为 100%[4,28,34]。

GeneXpert MTB RIF 分析是一种自动化的核酸扩增测试，需要操作员最少的时间和专业知识，可以在最短的 2 小时内产生结果。一项 meta 分析发现，与复合参考标准相比，肺外样本的敏感性和特异性分别为 81.2% 和 98% 以上。然而，GeneXpert 在检测液体样本（大多数数据来自 TPE 和脑脊液）时的灵敏度较低，与传统培养方法相似[21]。目前缺乏关于 GeneXpert MTB RIF 专门用于肠道和腹膜样本性能的良好数据。

3.4.7　免疫学

结核菌素皮肤试验仅在 50% 的 GI TB 诊断患者中呈阳性，在一些儿科人群中阳性率高达 80%～90%[20,57,73,83]。结核菌素皮肤试验阳性对活动性肺结核不是特异性的，可能代表潜在感染。

一项使用干扰素-γ 释放测定法（IGRA）诊断肠结核的 meta 分析中，阳性和阴性的似然比分别为 6.02 和 0.19[62]。鉴于 IGRA 无法区分活动性和潜伏性结核病感染，国际指南建议不要将其用于活动性结核病的诊断[86]。

3.5　治疗

3.5.1　药物治疗

对于以前没有接受过结核病治疗的未合并感染 HIV 的患者，6 个月的标准四联抗结核疗法已被证明与较长疗程一样有效[51]。对于证实或可能（由于当地流行病学、以前治疗过或治疗失败）耐药结核病的患者，根据当地或世界卫生组织的指南使用抗结核药物的组合治疗是合适的。新的抗分枝杆菌药物如贝达奎宁和地拉曼尼在治疗耐药性胃肠结核中的地位尚不明确，但它们很可能会起到一定的作用。一般说来，胃肠道和结核性腹膜炎的治疗方法与肺部结核非常相似，不同之处在于患者通常不会对他人构成感染风险。

随机对照试验没有解决常规使用类固醇在胃肠结核治疗中的作用，与现有出版物的数据相互矛盾[3,56]。类固醇不太可能在胃肠道疾病中提供治疗益处，我们不推荐常规使用。

3.5.2　外科治疗

随着有效的抗结核治疗的引入，手术在 GI TB 治疗中的作用在过去 50 年中发生了巨大的变化。治疗性外科手术现在主要保留给有急性手术紧急情况的患者，或者作为仅对药物治疗无效的患者的辅助治疗。在最近的成人队列中，15%～32%的患者需要手术[27,44]。在老年儿科队列中，有 7%～20%的患者需要手术干预，如因药物治疗不能治愈的梗阻而进行肠切除或狭窄成形术[57,83]。在一组钡检查有肠道狭窄证据的肠结核患者中，91%的患者接受了抗结核治疗，仅有 9%的患者需要手术治疗[5]。如果可能，最好采用补液和鼻胃减压的保守治疗方法，这样可以安全维持足够长的时间，从而使药物治疗有效。

3.6　预后

多达 3/4 的 GI TB 患者仅对药物治疗有反应[44]。然而，10%～15%的患者会发生部分肠梗阻，5%～10%的患者会出现完全性肠梗阻，4%～7%的患者会出现肠穿孔，2%～3%的患者会有需要干预的消化道出血，1%～2%的患者会出现瘘管[18,27,44,71]。3%的蛋白丢失性肠病和 2%的乳糜性腹水也被描述为儿科队列中的并发症[57]。报告的 GI TB 总死亡率差异很大，其中一些差异是由于未纳入经尸检诊断的患者造成的。据报道，儿科患儿的病死率为 3%～8%，其中出现肠穿孔的患儿病死率最高[52,57]。在成人中，报告的病死率从 5%到 50%不等，年龄较大、合并肝硬化和治疗延迟与较高的死亡可能性相关[12,15,16,25,44,51]。然而，这些数据来自世界不同地区在不同时间报道的不同研究，这些研究往往对 GI TB 的认识较少，缺乏确切的数据。所有的数据都必须非常谨慎地解读，没有考虑到诊断，很可能是病死率的最大驱动因素之一。

3.7　研究重点

最迫切的需要是对胃肠结核和结核性腹膜炎进行更好地诊断测试，对耐药结核进行更好地治疗,以及使用生物标志来早期预测那些有不良预后风险的患者。印度的一项研究确实显示了在粪便样本上使用 PCR 快速、非侵入诊断肠道结核的前景[61],但是还需要进一步的工作来验证这些发现[9],而且在过去 10 年中在这一领域没有明显的进展报告。据我们所知,Xpert MTB RIF 在疑似肠结核患者的粪便样本上的使用尚未进行调查。在肺部疾病的背景下,人们对结核病生物标志物很感兴趣[85],研究是否有任何生物标志物对 EPTB 或 GI TB 具有特异性将是有意义的。目前有一小部分结核病新药在研发,在耐药性不断增加的时代,人们对宿主导向的治疗越来越感兴趣[26]。此外,尽管最近出现了挫折[6,40],但人们对接种疫苗预防或控制结核病仍有很高的兴趣,但在未来 5 年内研制出一种有效的新疫苗是非常不可能的。

3.8 摘要

肠结核和结核性腹膜炎可出现非特异性症状或与胃肠道受影响部分相关的症状。克罗恩病是一种重要的鉴别诊断。患者可能不仅会出现在内科医师面前,还会出现通常不处理结核病的外科医师面前,因此需要多学科治疗。有许多诊断方法,但明确的诊断通常需要侵入性组织取样,这可能不是在所有环境或所有年龄段都容易获得的。标准的短程化疗对大多数患者来说应该是治愈的,只有少数有急性并发症(如梗阻)的患者需要手术。缺乏关于全球疾病负担的数据,而且由于重点放在能够传播感染的患者身上,因此很可能会被低估。医师必须有较高的临床经验指数,才能做出及时地诊断并制定最佳的治疗方案。这种情况迫切需要生物标志物。

参考文献

[1] Al Karawi M, Mohamed A, Yasawy M, et al. Protean manifestation of gastrointestinal tuberculosis: report on 130 patients. J Clin Gastroenterol. 1995; 20: 225-232.
[2] Almadi MA, Ghosh S, Aljebreen AM. Differentiating intestinal tuberculosis from Crohn's disease: a diagnostic challenge. Am J Gastroenterol. 2009; 104 (4): 1003-1012.
[3] Alrajhi AA, M A H, Al-Hokail A, et al. Corticosteroid treatment of peritoneal tuberculosis. Clin Infect Dis. 1998; 27: 52-56.

[4] Amarapurkar DN, Patel ND, Rane PS. Diagnosis of Crohn's disease in India where tuberculosis is widely prevalent. World J Gastroenterol. 2008; 14: 741-746.

[5] Anand BS, Nanda R, Sachdev GK. Response of tuberculous stricture to antituberculous treatment. Gut. 1988; 29: 62-69.

[6] Arnold C. Tuberculosis vaccine faces setbacks but optimism remains. Lancet Respir Med. 2013; 1: 13.

[7] Aston NO. Abdominal tuberculosis. World J Surg. 1997; 21: 492-499.

[8] Aston NO, de Costa AM. Abdominal tuberculosis. Br J Clin Pract. 1990; 44(2): 58-61, 63.

[9] Balamurugan R, Venkataraman S, John KR. PCR amplification of the IS 6110 insertion element of Mycobacterium tuberculosis in fecal samples from patients with intestinal tuberculosis. J Clin Microbiol. 2006; 44: 1884-1886.

[10] Baloch NA, Baloch MA, Baloch FA. A study of 86 cases of abdominal tuberculosis. J Surg Pakistan. 2008; 13: 3-5.

[11] Bastani B, Shariatzadeh MR, Dehdashti F. Tuberculous peritonitis-report of 30 cases and review of the literature. Q J Med. 1985; 549-557.

[12] Bhansali SK. Abdominal tuberculosis. Experiences with 300 cases. Am J Gastroenterol. 1977; 67: 324-337.

[13] Boudiaf M, Zidi SH, Soyer P, et al. Tuberculous colitis mimicking Crohn's disease: utility of computed tomography in the differentiation. Eur Radiol. 1998; 8: 1221-1223.

[14] Chen R, Chen Y, Liu L, et al. The role of F-FDG PET/CT in the evaluation of peritoneal thickening of undetermined origin. Medicine (Baltimore). 2016; 95: 1-8.

[15] Chow KM, Chow VCY, Hung LCT, et al. Tuberculous peritonitis-associated mortality is high among patients waiting for the results of mycobacterial cultures of ascitic fluid samples. Clin Infect Dis. 2002; 35: 409-413.

[16] Chow KM, Chow VCY, Szeto CC. Indication for peritoneal biopsy in tuberculous peritonitis. Am J Surg. 2003; 185: 567-573.

[17] Das K, Ghoshal UC, Dhali GK, et al. Crohn's disease in India: a multicenter study from a country where tuberculosis is endemic. Dig Dis Sci. 2009; 54: 1099-1107.

[18] Das P, Shukla HS. Clinical diagnosis of abdominal tuberculosis. Br J Surg. 1976; 63: 941-946.

[19] Debi U, Ravisankar V, Prasad KK, et al. Abdominal tuberculosis of the gastrointestinal tract: revisited. World J Gastroenterol. 2014; 20: 14831-14840.

[20] Delisle M, Seguin J, Zeilinski D, Moore DL. Paediatric abdominal tuberculosis in developed countries: case series and literature review. Arch Dis Child. 2015; 253-258.

[21] Denkinger CM, Schumacher SG, Boehme CC, et al. Xpert MTB/RIF assay for the diagnosis of extrapulmonary tuberculosis: a systematic review and meta-analysis. Eur Respir J. 2014; 44: 435-446.

[22] Dinler G, Sensoy G, Helek D, Kalayci AG. Tuberculous peritonitis in children: report of nine patients and review of the literature. World J Gastroenterol. 2008; 14: 7235-7239.

[23] Donoghue HD, Holton J. Intestinal tuberculosis. Curr Opin Infect Dis. 2009; 22: 490-496.

[24] Elkington PT, Ugarte-Gil CA, Friedland JS. Matrix metalloproteinases in tuberculosis. Eur Respir J. 2011; 38: 456-464.
[25] Fee MJ, Oo MM, Gabayan AE, et al. Abdominal tuberculosis in patients infected with the human immunodeficiency virus. Clin Infect Dis. 1995; 20: 938-944.
[26] Friedland JS. Targeting the inflammatory response in tuberculosis. N Engl J Med. 2014; 371: 1354-1356.
[27] Gan H, Mely M, Zhao J, Zhu L. An analysis of the clinical, endoscopic, and pathologic features of intestinal tuberculosis. J Clin Gastroenterol. 2016; 50: 470-475.
[28] Gan HT, Chen YQ, Ouyang Q, et al. Differentiation between intestinal tuberculosis and Crohn's disease in endoscopic biopsy specimens by polymerase chain reaction. Am J Gastroenterol. 2002; 97: 1446-1451.
[29] Gilinsky N, Marks I, Kottler R, Price S. Abdominal tuberculosis. South African Med J. 1983; 64: 849-857.
[30] Granet E. Intestinal tuberculosis. A clinical, roentgenological and pathological study of 2086 patients affected with pulmonary tuberculosis. Am J Dig Dis Nutr. 1934; 2: 209-214.
[31] Grange JM, Yates MD, de Kantor IN. Guidelines for speciation within the Mycobacterium tuberculosis complex. World Health Organisation. 1996; 2: 1-23.
[32] Grosset J. Mycobacterium tuberculosis in the extracellular compartment: an underestimated adversary. Antimicrob Agents Chemother. 2003; 47: 833-836.
[33] Ha HK, Jung JI, Lee MS, et al. CT differentiation of tuberculous peritonitis and peritoneal carcinomatosis. Am J Roentgenol. 1996; 167: 743-748.
[34] Hong KD, Il LS, Moon HY. Comparison between laparoscopy and noninvasive tests for the diagnosis of tuberculous peritonitis. World J Surg. 2011; 35: 2369-2375.
[35] Horvath KD, Whelan RL. Intestinal tuberculosis: return of an old disease. Am J Gastroenterol. 1998; 93: 692-696.
[36] Ihekwaba FN. Abdominal tuberculosis: a study of 881 cases. J R Coll Surg Edinb. 1993; 38: 293-295.
[37] Iliyasu Z, Babashani M. Prevalence and predictors of tuberculosis coinfection among HIV-seropositive patients attending the Aminu Kano Teaching Hospital, northern Nigeria. J Epidemiol. 2009; 19: 81-87.
[38] Jain SK, Jain S, Jain M, Yaduvanshi A. Esophageal tuberculosis: is it so rare? Report of 12 cases and review of the literature. Am J Gastroenterol. 2002; 97: 287-291.
[39] Joshi AR, Basantani AS, Patel TC. Role of CT and MRI in abdominal tuberculosis. Curr Radiol Rep. 2014; 2: 66.
[40] Kaufmann SHE, Lange C, Rao M, et al. Progress in tuberculosis vaccine development and host-directed therapies-a state of the art review. Lancet Respir Med. 2014; 2: 301-320.
[41] Keane J, Gershon S, Wise R, et al. Tuberculosis associated with infliximab, a tumor necrosis factor alpha-neutralizing agent. N Engl J Med. 2001; 345: 1098-1104.
[42] Keane W, Peterson P. Host defense mechanisms of the peritoneal cavity and continuous ambulatory peritoneal dialysis. Perit Dial Int. 1984; 11: 14-21.

[43] Kedar RP, Shah PP, Shivde RS, Malde HM. Sonographic findings in gastrointestinal and peritoneal tuberculosis. Clin Radiol. 1994; 49: 24-29.
[44] Khan R, Abid S, Jafri W, et al. Diagnostic dilemma of abdominal tuberculosis in non-HIV patients: an ongoing challenge for physicians. World J Gastroenterol. 2006; 12: 6371-6375.
[45] Klimach OE, Ormerod LP. Gastrointestinal tuberculosis: a retrospective review of 109 cases in a district general hospital. QJM. 1985; 56: 569-578.
[46] Lee YJ, Yang S-K, Byeon J-S, et al. Analysis of colonoscopic findings in the differential diagnosis between intestinal tuberculosis and Crohn's disease. Endoscopy. 2006; 38: 592-597.
[47] Limsrivilai J, Shreiner AB, Pongpaibul A, et al. Meta-analytic Bayesian model for differentiating intestinal tuberculosis from Crohn's disease. Am J Gastroenterol. 2017; 112: 415-427.
[48] Lora MH, Reimer-McAtee MJ, Gilman RH, et al. Evaluation of Microscopic Observation Drug Susceptibility (MODS) and the string test for rapid diagnosis of pulmonary tuberculosis in HIV/AIDS patients in Bolivia. BMC Infect Dis. 2015; 15: 222.
[49] Lugton IW. Mucosa-associated lymphoid tissues as sites for uptake, carriage and excretion of tubercle bacilli and other pathogenic mycobacteria. Immunol Cell Biol. 1999; 77: 364-372.
[50] Mahajan R, Simon EG, Chacko A, et al. Endoscopic ultrasonography in pediatric patients — experience from a tertiary care center in India. Indian J Gastroenterol. 2016; 35: 14-19.
[51] Makharia GK, Ghoshal UC, Ramakrishna BS, et al. Intermittent directly observed therapy for abdominal tuberculosis: a multicenter randomized controlled trial comparing 6 months versus 9 months of therapy. Clin Infect Dis. 2015; 61: 750-757.
[52] Malik R, Srivastava A, Yachha SK, et al. Childhood abdominal tuberculosis: disease patterns, diagnosis, and drug resistance. Indian J Gastroenterol. 2015; 34: 418-425.
[53] Mandal S, Bradshaw L, Anderson LF, et al. Investigating transmission of Mycobacterium bovis in the United Kingdom in 2005 to 2008. J Clin Microbiol. 2011; 49: 1943-1950.
[54] Manohar A, Haffejee AA, Pettengell KE. Symptoms and investigative findings in 145 patients with tuberculous peritonitis diagnosed by peritoneoscopy and biopsy over a five year period. Gut. 1990; 31: 1130-1132.
[55] Marshall JB. Tuberculosis of the gastrointestinal tract and peritoneum. Am J Gastroenterol. 1993; 88: 989-999.
[56] McGowan JE, Chesney PJ, Crossley KB, LaForce FM. Guidelines for the use of systemic glucocorticosteroids in the management of selected infections. Jounal Infect Dis. 1992; 165: 1-13.
[57] Millar AJW, Rode H, Cywes S. Abdominal tuberculosis in children-surgical management. Pediatr Surg Int. 1990; 5: 392-396.
[58] Moore DAJ, Evans CAW, Gilman RH, et al. Microscopic-observation drug-

susceptibility assay for the diagnosis of TB. N Engl J Med. 2006; 355: 1539-1550.
[59] Muller B, Durr S, Alonso S, et al. Zoonotic mycobacterium bovis-induced tuberculosis in humans. Emerg Infect Dis. 2013; 19: 899-908.
[60] Nafeh MA, Medhat A, Abdul-Hameed AG, et al. Tuberculous peritonitis in Egypt: the value of laparoscopy in diagnosis. Am J Trop Med Hyg. 1992; 47: 470-477.
[61] Nakamura M, Niwa Y, Ohmiya N, et al. Small bowel tuberculosis diagnosed by the combination of video capsule endoscopy and double balloon enteroscopy. Eur J Gastroenterol Hepatol. 2007; 19: 595-598.
[62] Ng SC, Hirai HW, Tsoi KKF, et al. Systematic review with meta-analysis: accuracy of interferon-gamma releasing assay and anti-Saccharomyces cerevisiae antibody in differentiating intestinal tuberculosis from Crohn's disease in Asians. J Gastroenterol Hepatol. 2014; 29: 1664-1670.
[63] Ong CWM, Elkington PT, Brilha S, et al. Neutrophil-derived MMP-8 drives AMPK-dependent matrix destruction in human pulmonary tuberculosis. PLoS Pathog. 2015; 11: 1-21.
[64] Palmer KR, Patil DH, Basran GS, et al. Abdominal tuberculosis in urban Britain — a common disease. Gut. 1985; 26: 1296-1305.
[65] Peto HM, Pratt RH, Harrington TA, et al. Epidemiology of extrapulmonary tuberculosis in the United States, 1993-2006. Clin Infect Dis. 2009; 49: 1350-1357.
[66] Porter JC, Friedland JS, Freedman AR. Tuberculous bronchoesophageal fistulae in patients infected with the human immunodeficiency virus: three case reports and review. Clin Infect Dis. 1994; 19: 954-957.
[67] Poyrazoglu OK, Timurkaan M, Yalniz M, et al. Clinical review of 23 patients with tuberculous peritonitis: presenting features and diagnosis. J Dig Dis. 2008; 9: 170-174.
[68] Pulimood AB, Amarapurkar DN, Ghoshal U, et al. Differentiation of Crohn's disease from intestinal tuberculosis in India in 2010. World J Gastroenterol. 2011; 17: 433-443.
[69] Puri R, Khaliq A, Kumar M, et al. Esophageal tuberculosis: role of endoscopic ultrasound in diagnosis. Dis Esophagus. 2012; 25: 102-106.
[70] Ramakrishnan L. Revisiting the role of the granuloma in tuberculosis. Nat Rev Immunol. 2012; 12: 352-366.
[71] Ramesh J, Banait GS, Ormerod LP. Abdominal tuberculosis in a district general hospital: a retrospective review of 86 cases. QJM. 2008; 101: 189-195.
[72] Rodwell TC, Moore M, Moser KS, et al. Tuberculosis from Mycobacterium bovis in binational communities, United States. Emerg Infect Dis. 2008; 14: 909-916.
[73] Sanai FM, Bzeizi KI. Systematic review: tuberculous peritonitis-presenting features, diagnostic strategies and treatment. Aliment Pharmacol Ther. 2005; 22: 685-700.
[74] Sandgren A, Hollo V, van der Werf MJ. Extrapulmonary tuberculosis in the European union and European economic area, 2002 to 2011. Eur Surveill. 2013; 18(12): 1-9.
[75] Sarin R, Mehta S, Sarin J. Punch biopsy of the peritoneum. Br Med J. 1961; 1:

100 - 102.
[76] Shakil AO, Korula J, Kanel GC, et al. Diagnostic features of tuberculous peritonitis in the absence and presence of chronic liver disease: a case control study. Am J Med. 1996; 100: 179 - 185.
[77] Shao H, Yang ZG, Deng W, et al. Tuberculosis versus lymphoma in the abdominal lymph nodes: a comparative study using contrast-enhanced MRI. Eur J Radiol. 2012; 81: 2513 - 2517.
[78] Sharma MP, Bhatia V. Abdominal tuberculosis. Indian J Med Res. 2004; 120: 305 - 315.
[79] Shukla HS, Bhatiat S, Naitrani YP, et al. Peritoneal biopsy for diagnosis of abdominal tuberculosis. Postgrad Med J. 1982; 58: 226 - 228.
[80] Singh MM, Bhargava AN, Jain KP. Tuberculous peritonitis. An evaluation of pathogenetic mechanisms, diagnostic procedures and therapeutic measures. N Engl J Med. 1969; 281: 1091 - 1094.
[81] Suri S, Gupta S, Suri R. Computed tomography in abdominal tuberculosis. Br J Radiol. 1999; 72: 92 - 98.
[82] Talwani R, Horvath JA. Tuberculous peritonitis in patients undergoing continuous ambulatory peritoneal dialysis: case report and review. Clin Infect Dis. 2000; 31: 70 - 75.
[83] Talwar S, Talwar R, Chowdhary B, Prasad P. Abdominal tuberculosis in children: an Indian experience. J Trop Pediatr. 2000; 46: 368 - 370.
[84] Tandon HD, Prakash a. Pathology of intestinal tuberculosis and its distinction from Crohn's disease. Gut. 1972; 13: 260 - 269.
[85] Wallis RS, Maeurer M, Mwaba P, et al. Tuberculosis-advances in development of new drugs, treatment regimens, host-directed therapies, and biomarkers. Lancet Infect Dis. 2016; 16: e34 - 46.
[86] World Health Organisation. Use of tuberculosis interferon-gamma release assays (IGRAs) in low- and middle-income countries: policy statement; 2011.

4 肝胆脾结核

久姆胡尔·阿尔图克和汉尼菲·杰姆·居尔

4.1 肝胆结核

肝受累可能是由于器官受累所致，也可能是由各种感染源引起的原发性感染，或者是作为多系统疾病的一个组成部分。临床症状通常与其他临床症状相似。结核病是发展中国家的一种常见疾病，在发达国家，特别是在HIV患者和移民人口中，结核病的发病率呈上升趋势[1,2]。肝结核是一种罕见的器官受累，是结核分枝杆菌引起的最常见的感染性临床疾病之一。肝胆结核的定义是指肝胆受累，包括肝、胆管或肝胆系统的其他器官孤立受累。结核性肝损害的临床病程多种多样，常用来描述肝胆系统的损害。结核可表现为结核性假瘤、结核性胆管炎、结核性肝脓肿和结核杆菌感染性肝炎[3-7]。

4.1.1 流行病学特征

结核病是一种常见病，发病率和病死率都很高，特别是在不发达或发展中国家的人口中。在世界范围内，估计有20亿人患有潜伏性结核病，每年新发现700万～800万病例。尽管有有效的治疗，但仍有200万人死于这种疾病，特别是在不发达国家[8]。虽然结核主要累及肺部，但肺外病变的发生率为15%～20%，可累及任何部位身体器官[9]。腹部结核并不常见，但约占EPTB病例的3.5%。在其他类型的腹部结核中，肝结核非常罕见。它通常见于播散性肺结核病例[8,10,11]。原发性肝胆结核占所有结核病例的1%[1,12,13]。在腹腔内结核中，6%～38%的患者在诊断时就有活动性肺结核的表现。

肝结核在亚洲国家较为常见,肝胆结核在菲律宾人中较为常见。这一事实还没有得到明确的解释,但观察结果支持菲律宾人可能有结核病的种族易感性[1]。在世界范围内的文献中,许多病例报道了局限性肝结核,特别是作为菲律宾患者梗阻性黄疸的病因[15-18]。由于缺乏特异性的临床表现,也没有特异性的诊断试验来帮助诊断肝结核,只有在手术后对切除的组织进行组织病理学检查后才能做出明确的诊断。在尸检中,高达90%的肺结核相关死亡病例可以看到肝受累[11]。

肝胆结核在男性中的发病率是女性的两倍。虽然具体的年龄组还没有定义,但一项研究报告称,在11~50岁的年龄组中观察到的频率更高[19]。

4.1.2 发病机制

肝结核感染是通过在肝内形成肉芽肿来限制疾病的发生,与结核杆菌进入的途径无关。结核杆菌可以通过血源性途径到达肝,因为它可以从原发肺部感染部位通过肝动脉传播到肝,或者通过门静脉从胃肠系统传播到肝。结核性淋巴结破裂后,感染也可能通过淋巴途径传播到肝[20,21]。这种疾病的血源性传播比通过淋巴途径或门静脉传播更为频繁。在粟粒型肺结核中,间歇性发作时,血源性扩散会导致肝中结核小病灶的数量增加。

在肝结核中,肉芽肿可以是干酪性的,也可以是非干酪性的。在粟粒性结核中,在肝脏的多个小结核病灶中可观察到中央干酪和纤维素样坏死,周边可见直径可变的上皮细胞冠状突起,内嵌有朗汉斯巨细胞。肉芽肿性结节周围有大量淋巴细胞。结核性肉芽肿最常见于门脉周围区域。在粟粒型结核或局部结核中,原发性结核复合体合并形成结核瘤。它们形成直径1~4 cm的结节。内含钙化是结核球的典型特征,它们最终会被包裹起来。这些结节有时是血源性扩散的来源。

肝胆结核根据其发病机制特点可表现为多种临床表现[2,9]:

被肺结核附带。在活动性肺结核死亡的患者中,有25%~50%的人尸检发现肝受累。

粟粒型结核(由于结核杆菌的血源性传播)导致肝多发性肉芽肿。这是最流行和最常见的肝结核形式,据报道,在所有死于肺结核的患者中,有50%~80%会出现这种情况[11]。

肉芽肿性肝炎。结核球融合,结节大小为1~4 cm。患者有不明原因的发热、黄疸、肝大、碱性磷酸酶升高,以及其他肝功能检查异常。肝影像学可以显示正常的表现,也可以观察到非特异性异常。这时腹腔镜检查是有用的,可以发现肝表面不规则的白色干酪样结节。在这些病变的活检材料中,可见干酪样肉芽肿。接种卡介苗后可能会发生肝多发性肉芽肿伴肉芽肿性肝炎,特别是在免疫功能低下的个体中。

结节性疾病。这些病变在肝以单发或多发性病变的形式发展,可视为低密度、非扩张性病变,伴或不伴周围扩张。观察这种类型的结构需要与淋巴瘤、真菌感染和转移进行鉴别诊断。诊断应通过影像引导下细针穿刺活检确诊。

结核性肝脓肿。肝的结核性脓肿非常罕见。临床和影像学表现与化脓性和阿米巴性脓肿相似。诊断是通过从脓肿的抽吸物中培养结核杆菌。

肝胆管(导管)疾病。这些患者因胆管受累而表现为梗阻性黄疸。胆管受累可能是由于结核杆菌弥漫性累及肝内胆管,或由于结核淋巴结肿大对胆管的压迫。ERCP显示多处肝内胆道狭窄,并显示扩张和扩张区域,有助于区分胆管癌和硬化性胆管炎。胆道狭窄可发生在肝门区或广泛分布于远端胆管,其特征是肝内胆管扩张[2]。

4.1.3 临床特征

肝胆结核的临床表现与肝外疾病相似,是非特异性的,肝受累通常是无症状的。在各种病例系列中,非特异性腹痛和右上腹痛被报道为最常见的症状。常见症状和体征如下[3,12,19,21]:

右上腹疼痛	65%～87%
非特异性症状(发热、厌食、体重减轻)	55%～90%
非特异性腹痛	50%
黄疸	20%～35%
肝大	70%～96%
脾大	25%～55%

由于EPTG通常是这样的,患者常会出现不明原因的发热。临床症状中还包括其他一些不适,例如厌食和体重减轻。随着病情的进展,最初的非特异性腹痛在整个腹部,然后局限于右上腹[3,22]。它发生在55%～90%的患者中。

临床表现提示急性胆囊炎或胆绞痛可表现在孤立的胆管结核中。黄疸的存在提示胆道受累，生化检查结果可能与肝外胆道梗阻相似。黄疸或胆管狭窄是由以下因素引起的，包括门静脉肝淋巴结压迫胆管、胆管周围炎症，直接累及胆管上皮，以及位于胆管内的结核性肉芽肿破裂[23]。肉芽肿累及肝内胆道梗阻可发展为粟粒型结核的一部分。胆管结核可发展为胆管扩张并伴有广泛的肝管狭窄。具有这些病状的患者表现出无痛性黄疸和体重减轻，通常与胰腺癌或胆管癌相似。只有45%的黄疸患者伴有腹痛[18]。

结核性肝脓肿症状无特异性，以发热、腹痛为主，其他发现包括体重减轻和黄疸[12,18,21,24,25]。孤立性胰腺结核的临床表现可能与胰腺肿瘤相似。

肝大是最常见的发现，在70%～96%的患者中观察到，类似于孤立的肝肿瘤或肝脓肿[18,21]。在大约一半的类似肝癌的病例中，肝脏呈坚硬结节状，因此，临床表现与肿瘤相同。在36%的肝脓肿的病例中也有类似的情况。25%～55%的患者有脾大[3,18]。

4.1.4　诊断

由于肝胆疾病的症状多种多样，诊断具有挑战性，因此需要高水平的证据[26]。生化检查表明肝结核的存在并不具有特异性。虽然包括天冬氨酸转氨酶、丙氨酸氨基转移酶、碱性磷酸酶、γ-谷氨酰转肽酶、总蛋白和白蛋白/球蛋白比值在内的肝功能检测在30%～80%的患者中较高，但它们对肝胆结核的诊断没有特异性或病因学意义[18]。血清碱性磷酸酶不成比例的高水平是一个支持点，与肝浸润的过程相一致。在肝结核中，转氨酶的水平高于碱性磷酸酶（ALP）。然而，在胆道或门静脉受累的病例中，ALP较高。与梗阻相关的实质性疾病相比，肝外结核患者的胆红素水平较高。胆红素、胰岛素受体和白蛋白水平的改变是肝衰竭进展的证据[9]。

虽然在肺结核患者的晚期诊断过程中可以发现肝结核，但大约75%的患者有支持肺结核的异常胸片[9,25]。影像学技术在肝胆结核的诊断中起着关键作用。在腹部X线片上观察到肝上的钙化有时见于局部肝结核。超声检查（USG）不仅能提供肝胆结核的诊断，还能检测出晚期临床体征，如LAP、腹水和积液[27-30]。在超声检查中，结核性肝脓肿和假瘤性肝结核表现为单个或多个复杂的肿块和低回声病灶，没有明显的壁，很难与癌症区分开。CT 和 MRI 有助于结核球或结核性肝脓肿的诊断。肝结核球由于干酪样坏死，表现为非增生性中央低密度病灶，周围稍形成边缘，与周围肉芽组织相对应。然而，这些发现也见于坏死性肿瘤，如肝细胞癌和转移性癌[31,32]。肝钙化也可以通过 CT 扫描显示出来。通过 USG 和 CT 引导下穿刺和活检获得的结果是诊断的重要因素[33]。内镜超声造影（EUS）是胰腺和胆道病变随访的常规方法，可从这些病变部位取样[34,35]。这些方法也可用于肝病变。USG 和 CT 引导下的活检是首选，因为 EUS 更具侵袭性，而且有经验的人员有限[36]。MR 在肝胆结核的诊断中没有提供额外的优势。

在肝胆结核中，即使在取样了相关组织之后，仍然难以做出诊断。显微镜检查、培养、组织学、ELISA 和 PCR 在进行诊断时都非常重要[37,38]。然而，诊断率因相关样本的可用性和这些检测的可用性而异。对干酪性肉芽肿的组织病理学证实，对 ZN-染色的活检标本的直接检查或对抗酸杆菌的培养都可以对局部或弥漫性肝结核的明确诊断。其目的应是直接或通过培养证实肝中结核杆菌的存在。肉芽肿的大小通常为 1~2 mm，但也有大到 12 cm 的结核球报道。在 80%~100% 的病例中，肝结核可形成上皮样肉芽肿。布鲁菌病、球孢子菌病和霍奇金病在鉴别诊断中也应考虑，因为在这些疾病的病程中存在肉芽肿[39-41]。在对几个病例进行的肝活检中，33%~100% 的病例显示，干酪样是结核性肉芽肿的特征性表现[12,25,42,43]。在肝结核病例的活检和穿刺标本中抗酸杆菌的检出率为 7%~59%[12,25,44]。结核培养阳性可确诊，然而，培养提供阳性结果的比率为 10%[42]。将培养物和镜检结果相结合时，诊断率上升到 30%~50%[9]。

T-SPOT 或 QuantiFERON 结核菌检测用于检测干扰素-γ 的存在，这种干扰素是由外周单个核细胞对结核分枝杆菌的特异性抗原产生的。近年来，它在结核病的诊断中得到了较高的应用，灵敏度可达 70%~90%，比结核菌素皮肤试验更具特异性[45]。在分子生物学方法中，PCR 在大多数肝结核性肉芽肿患者中具有病因学意义。虽然这些研究在确诊肺结核患者（干酪样肉芽肿患者）中确定了 100% 的阳性率，但据报道，在肝胆结核的预诊断患者中成功率为 78%[46]。

在影像学技术和实验室检查未能确诊的情况下，腹腔镜检查可对有临床表现的肝结核做出诊断和鉴别诊断。腹腔镜检查可以检查病变并取样相关材料[3,18]。在胆管结核的诊断中，特别是梗阻性黄疸的病例中，ERCP 的应用为诊断和治疗提供了有价值的贡献[42]。

诊断方法的灵敏度[1]	
肝功能受损	30%～80%
胸片异常	75%
组织病理学评价	
上皮样肉芽肿形成	80%～100%
干酪性坏死	33%～100%
抗酸的细菌	60%
PCR	88%

4.1.5 治疗

除治疗时间不同外,肝结核的治疗与其他临床肺外结核相同。按照世卫组织建议,传统四药抗结核治疗仍然是治疗的基石[9]。治疗由 4 种药物联合组成:异烟肼[5 mg/(kg·d)]、利福平[10 mg/(kg·d)]、吡嗪酰胺[30 mg/(kg·d)]和乙胺丁醇[20 mg/(kg·d)]。一般来说,4 种药物治疗最初的治疗时间为 2~4 个月,然后是异烟肼和利福平治疗 6~12 个月。虽然 6 个月的疗程对于抗结核治疗来说通常是足够的,但由于多重耐药杆菌或肝毒性药物的存在,需要替代方案。尤其是异烟肼可能会导致特征性的继发性肝损害,而且可能是致命的。密切随访患者可以防止这种死亡。美国胸科学会建议密切监测血清 ALT 水平,特别是在饮酒患者,使用其他肝毒性药物的患者,HIV 阳性患者,基线 ALT 水平异常的患者,既往有肝病、病毒性肝炎和与异烟肼相关的肝炎病史的患者,孕妇和产后 3 个月内的患者[31]。在标准的抗结核治疗中,一些研究表明,当利福平和 INH 联合使用时,67% 的患者的腹痛和发热得到缓解,食欲和体重增加,肝恢复正常大小,病死率显著降低[12]。

在对结核性肝脓肿进行经皮引流和穿刺抽吸的同时,使用抗结核药物至少 6 个月可提高治疗成功率[5,31,38,39,47]。由于诊断困难,特别是在结节性肝结核的病例中,并且由于病变的恶性潜能,肝切除术可能被认为是一种替代治疗[48]。如果梗阻性黄疸患者在抗结核治疗的基础上加用 ERCP 和支架治疗,临床病程无明显改善,可行经皮胆管引流或外科减压术。

肝结核的累计病死率为 15%～42%,肝功能衰竭引起的死亡很少见[12]。继发于肝硬化的呼吸衰竭和静脉曲张出血是有其他原因[18]。预后不良的危险因素有：
- 血型播散型肺结核
- 同时使用类固醇
- 年龄小于 20 岁
- 恶病质
- HIV 阳性
- 肝硬化
- 肝衰竭

4.1.6 并发症

结核性结节穿透胆管可引起胆道结核，导致受影响区域狭窄[23]。这些结核性结节中结核杆菌和干酪样坏死的存在可能导致肝腔的形成。因此，结核性脓肿、生长性脓肿或假肿瘤性肝结核的鉴别诊断变得更加困难[18]。肝胆结核罕见的临床表现是结核淋巴结压迫导致门静脉高压并发静脉曲张出血。结核性假性肝硬化可能是由于在恢复过程中出现少量多发结节的碎屑或弥漫性播散，然而，它不是作为主要肝功能障碍的恢复过程的后遗症而发展的。慢性肺结核可发生肝淀粉样变性和肝功能障碍[49]。大量粟粒扩散到肝脏可能导致急性肝功能衰竭，以及感染性休克伴发多器官衰竭[50]。

4.2 脾结核

科利（Coley）在 1846 年首次将脾结核描述为由于结核引起的继发性脾大，包括仅局限于其他器官累及或者没有任何其他器官的累及[51]。除少数病例外，脾结核相当罕见[52,53]。脾结核主要发生在免疫功能低下的患者中，通常是在结核分枝杆菌阳性病灶的血行播散后发生的。作为粟粒型结核的一种表现，它排在肺和肝受累之后的第三位[54-57]。孤立性脾结核是相当罕见的，特别是在免疫能力正常的患者中[57-60]。EPTB 在发展中国家仍然是一个公共卫生问题。EPTB 的常见形式有结核性淋巴结炎、结核性胸膜炎、结核性关节、结核性腹膜炎、结核性心包炎、结核性脑膜炎和粟粒型结核等[61-63]。

4.2.1 流行病学

在20世纪70年代结核病的发病率稳步下降之后，发达国家的结核病发病率在80年代艾滋病暴发后也呈上升趋势[63,64]。虽然肺结核是最常见的结核形式，但近年来播散性和肺外结核的发病率有所增加[65]。70％的结核病和HIV感染患者可见肺外疾病侵犯骨关节、大脑和肾[40]。15％～20％的结核病例属于肺外，其中3％～11％属于腹部[66,67]。腹部结核见于回盲部、肛门直肠区、淋巴结和腹膜。已有免疫功能低下的肺结核患者出现静脉血栓和脾脓肿的报道。然而，在免疫功能正常的患者中，孤立性脾静脉血栓形成和多发性脾脓肿是相当罕见的[61]。在一些病例中，脾结核的发生率为8％，小结节受累的发生率为5％[52]。几项尸检报告显示，脾结核的发病率很低（0.14％～0.7％），且这些病例通常与败血症有关[68]。

根据世卫组织2016年全球结核病报告，结核病仍然是十大最常见的病死和发病原因之一，甚至超过了HIV感染造成的病死率。根据该报告，2015年，全世界有1 040万人感染了结核病，其中140万人死于该种疾病。根据世界卫生组织的监测数据，结核病是非洲的一个主要问题。在同一份报告中，全世界所有新发病例中，据报告26％发生在非洲，年发病率为275/10万，是全球年发病率142/10万的近两倍[69]。在HIV-1感染CD4计数低的患者中，脾结核或肝结核可能是结核病的最初临床表现。诊断是困难的，经常会被漏诊。

脾结核发生的危险因素如下[70,71]：
- 免疫抑制（HIV阳性、系统性红斑狼疮、类固醇使用者）；
- 化脓性感染的存在和传播；
- 脾异常；
- 既往脾外伤史；
- 镰状细胞贫血；
- 其他血红蛋白疾病；
- 具有免疫能力的患者体内其他部位感染结核分枝杆菌；
- 存在胃脾瘘[72]。

4.2.2 临床特点

在文献中,脾结核最初的特征性临床表现是不明原因的发热[74,75]。除了最常见的发热症状(82.3%)外,其他症状包括疲劳和体重减轻(44.12%)、脾大(13.2%～100%)、自发性脾破裂、脾功能亢进、门脉高压伴或不伴消化道出血,以及快速进展的暴发型形式[66,76,77]。发热、恶病质、出血和脓毒症的快速进展是暴发性疾病的表现形式[77]。很少情况下,患者可能会没有症状,可能仍未得到诊断。疼痛并不常见[54]。血液学异常,细胞计数减少和红细胞增多在病例报告中被报道[78]。不明确和非特异性的临床症状以及缺乏特征性的放射学表现,导致对孤立性结核的诊断存在不确定性[55,63,70]。

文献中已有脾结核的病例报道。其中一篇描述了一个患者以很快疲倦、虚弱、呼吸困难和盗汗为主诉。体格检查发现脾大。超声检查为低回声,CT检查为低密度病变。此外,胸部和腹部内淋巴结病(lymphadenopathies,LAP)也在CT中被发现。考虑为慢性淋巴增生综合征;然而,令人惊讶的是,在组织病理学检查中,诊断为脾结核[79]。

脓肿形成在脾结核中很少见,最常见于 HIV 阳性患者[61]。深静脉血栓形成虽然非常罕见,但尤其是在广泛且严重的结核病例中应予以考虑[80]。与结核相关的血栓事件可发生在不同部位,如肝静脉或脑静脉窦。与其他传染病一样,结核病可通过多种机制引起血栓形成[61],包括:

- 局部侵犯
- 静脉压迫
- 高凝状态

纤维蛋白溶解受损、血浆纤维蛋白原增加、抗凝血酶Ⅲ水平降低和活性血小板增多,都会导致结核 DVT 的发生[61]。

非创伤性自发性脾破裂非常罕见,但却是危及生命的急症。如果不及时诊断和治疗,最终会导致 100% 的病例死亡。在自发性脾破裂的病因学中,恶性肿瘤居首位,占 30.3%,感染次之,占 27.3%。这两种病因同时出现的情况相当罕见。在文献中,报道了一例急性髓系白血病患者并发脾结核的自发性脾破裂患者[81]。

这些发现包括患者的临床情况恶化,现有病变的进展,或治疗中出现新的病变被定义为矛盾反应。矛盾反应通常与肺部受累、淋巴结炎和发热等炎症表现相关。抗生素治疗对杆菌的迅速破坏导致微生物成分大量释放，导致炎症反应增加。持久的分枝杆菌抗原可引起超敏反应。临床可能会忽视一种矛盾的反应，导致结核病患者因误诊而终止治疗。此外，这种自相矛盾的反应本身也受到限制，因此并不是所有的病例都需要类固醇治疗[70]。

4.2.3　诊断

这些患者的 PPD 通常呈阳性，然而，在该病流行的国家、免疫功能低下的患者和接种了卡介苗的患者中，它并不可靠。PCR 更敏感、更具特异性，可以识别微生物的亚型。在这些病例中，腹部超声（USG）是一种无创且经济实惠的检查方法，可以显示粟粒型结核、结节性结核、结核性脾脓肿、钙化结核性病变或它们的组合[73]。结核球表现为多发高回声病灶，其边界以后方扩张为界。当这些病变出现时，以下疾病包括淋巴瘤、急性白血病、血管瘤、转移和真菌感染应考虑在鉴别诊断[57]。腹部 CT 在确定脏器受累方面优于腹部 USG，可显示除脾结核外的多个分界性低密度病灶（8.21）。CT 可显示均匀的脾肿大或结核球，表现为非扩张性的均匀低密度[53,77]。孤立性巨大脾肿大的鉴别诊断应考虑囊肿、血肿、真菌感染、脓肿、梗死、淋巴瘤、血管性或转移性肿瘤等临床症状[70]。虽然没有典型的形态学表现，但脾的细、粗针穿刺活检是有价值的，组织病理学诊断很重要（敏感性 88%，特异性 100%）[54,57,67,70,77]。通过显微镜检查确定了病变的组织学类型以及结核性病变的分期，可以对其他肉芽肿性病变和其他混杂的放射学性病变如淋巴瘤进行鉴别诊断。福尔马林组织固定和二甲苯处理降低了抗酸染色（acid-fast staining，AFS）的敏感性，导致假阴性结果。福尔马林固定和石蜡包埋的组织在抗酸显微镜下无法识别结核杆菌。对这些病例的组织标本进行实时 PCR 检测，其敏感性高于 AFS。核心针穿刺活检（core needle biopsy，CNB）在脾病理诊断中具有较高的诊断价值，与细针抽吸细胞学（fine needle aspiration cytology，FNAC）相比，对脾病变的定性诊断准确率更高。含有上皮样细胞和朗汉斯巨细胞的肉芽肿以及典型的病例证实为结核性感染[70]。目前用于明确诊断的是参考培养试验[69]。在不明原因发热伴脾大的情况下，应注意结核。在组织病理学上检测干酪样肉芽肿将具有病理意义。当不能用非侵入性方法进行诊断时，腹腔镜检查可作为指征，然而，脾切除术应考虑为诊断的最后努力。脾脏脓肿需要引流，因为这些病例的放射诊断方法是不够的。通过显微镜检查很少可能检测到抗酸细菌；因此，分子方法仍然是快速诊断结核病的有价值的方法[63]。

4.2.4 治疗

抗结核治疗是治疗的首选[53,66,76,77]。三联或四联治疗应维持至少 12 个月。除了一些罕见的临床情况外，脾切除术是一种无效的治疗方法[61,66,77]。

脾切除术适应证[53,55,56,61]：
- 抗结核治疗失败，存在血细胞减少或红细胞增多；
- 脾结核合并 GIS 继发门静脉高压出血；
- 经皮脓肿引流失败；
- 多发性脾脓肿；
- 存在脾破裂。

抗结核治疗应维持到脾切除术后。USG 和 CT 成像可以用来评估治疗的成功程度[78]。MRI 和 PET 成像在确定脾脏病变的活动性以及识别其他活动性和纤维化瘢痕方面是有用的[82]。

由于脾脏静脉血栓形成的病例很少见，因此评价抗凝治疗效果的对照研究目前还缺乏。不推荐对无症状患者进行抗凝治疗[83]。抗凝治疗的潜在好处是可以防止门静脉、门静脉后和门静脉侧支静脉血栓的形成。孤立性内脏静脉血栓的鉴别诊断应考虑结核。抗结核治疗应作为辅助治疗，特别是在累及肠系膜的情况下[61]。

4.2.5 并发症

如果脾结核诊断延误，抗结核治疗不及时，术后可能出现颅内结核脓肿、肺结核等并发症。可以看到全身性播散；然而，开始抗结核治疗将有助于恢复[71]。

参考文献

肝胆肺结核

[1] Chaudhary P. Hepatobiliary tuberculosis. Ann Gastroenterol. 2014；27(3)：207-217.

- [2] Khuroo MS, Khuroo MS, Diseases H. In: Guerrant RL, Walker DH, Weller PF, editors. Trop infect dis: Princ, path Prac. 3rd ed. Philadelphia: Saunders; 2011. p. 975-981.
- [3] Alvarez SZ. Hepatobiliary tuberculosis. J Gastroenterol Hepatol. 1998; 13: 833-839.
- [4] Chong VH. Hepatobiliary tuberculosis: a review of presentations and outcome. South Med J. 2008; 101: 356-361.
- [5] Goh KL, Pathmanathan R, Chang IW, Wong NW. Tuberculous liver abscess. J Trop Med. 1987; 90: 255-257.
- [6] Weinberg JJ, Cohen P, Malhotra R. Primary tuberculous liver abscess associated with human immunodeficiency virus. Tubercle. 1988; 69: 145-147.
- [7] Spiegel CT, Tuozon CD. Tuberculous liver abscess. Tubercle. 1984; 65: 127-31.
- [8] Chong VH, Lim KS. Hepatobiliary tuberculosis. Singap Med J. 2010; 51(9): 744-751.
- [9] Evans RP, Mourad MM, Dvorkin L, Bramhall SR. Hepatic and intra-abdominal tuberculosis: 2016 update. Curr Infect Dis Rep. 2016; 18(12): 45.
- [10] Amarapurkar DN, Patel ND, Amarapurkar AD. Hepatobiliary tuberculosis in western India. Indian J Pathol Microbiol. 2008; 51(2): 175.
- [11] Morris E. Tuberculosis of the liver. Am Rev Tuberc. 1930; 22: 585-592.
- [12] Essop AR, Posen JA, Hodkinson JH, Segal I, Tuberculosis h. A clinical review of 96 cases. Q J Med. 1984; 53(4): 465-477.
- [13] Tai W-C, Kuo C-M, Lee C-H, Chuah S-K, Huang C-C, Hu T-H, et al. Liver tuberculosis in Southern Taiwan: 15-years clinical experience. Intern Med Chi. 2008; 19: 410-417.
- [14] Hulnick DH, Megibow AJ, Naidich DP, Hilton Z, Cho KC, Balthazar EJ. Abdominal tuberculosis: CT evaluation. Radiology. 1985; 157(1): 199-204.
- [15] Bristowe JS. On the connection between abscess of the liver and gastrointestinal ulceration. Trans Pathol Soc. 1958; 9: 241.
- [16] Fan ST, Ng IOL, Choi TK, Lai ECS. Tuberculosis of the bile duct. A rare cause of biliary stricture. Am J Gastroenterol. 1989; 84: 413-414.
- [17] Gallinger S, Strasberg SM, Marcus HI, Brunton J. Local hepatic tuberculosis, the cause of a painful hepatic mass: case report and review of literature. Can J Surg. 1986; 29: 451-452.
- [18] Alvarez SZ, Carpio R. Hepatobiliary tuberculosis. Dig Dis Sci. 1983; 28: 193-200.
- [19] Oliva A, Duarte B, Jonasson O, Nadimpalli V. The nodular form of local hepatic tuberculosis. J Clin Gastroenterol. 1990; 12: 166.
- [20] Terry RB, Gunnar RM. Primary miliary tuberculosis of the liver. J Am Med Assoc. 1957; 164(2): 150-157.
- [21] Hersch C. Tuberculosis of the liver. S Afr Med J. 1964; 38: 857.
- [22] Hickey N, McNulty JG, Osborne H, Finucane J. Acute hepatobiliary tuberculosis a report of two cases and a review of the literature. Eur Radiol. 1999; 9(5): 886-889.
- [23] Kok KY, Yapp SK. Tuberculosis of the bile duct: a rare cause of obstructive jaundice. J Clin Gastroenterol. 1999; 29: 161-164.
- [24] Dey J, Gautam H, Venugopal S, Porwal C, Mirdha BR, Gupta N, Singh UB.

Tuberculosis as an etiological factor in liver abscess in adults. Tuberc Res Treat. 2016; 2016: 8479456.

[25] Maharaj B, Leary WP, Pudifin DJ. A prospective study of hepatic tuberculosis in 41 black patients. Quart. J Med. 1987; 63: 517-522.

[26] Burke KA, Patel A, Jayaratnam A, Thiruppathy K, Snooks SJ. Diagnosing abdominal tuberculosis in the acute abdomen. Int J Surg. 2014; 12(5): 494-499.

[27] von Hahn T, Bange F-C, Westhaus S, Rifai K, Attia D, Manns M, et al. Ultrasound presentation of abdominal tuberculosis in a German tertiary care center. Scand J Gastroenterol. 2014; 49(2): 184-190.

[28] Atzori S, Vidili G, Delitala G. Usefulness of ultrasound in the diagnosis of peritoneal tuberculosis. J Infect Develop Countries. 2012; 6(12): 886-890.

[29] Goblirsch S, Bahlas S, Ahmed M, Brunetti E, Wallrauch C, Heller T. Ultrasound findings in cases of extrapulmonary TB in patients with HIV infection in Jeddah, Saudi Arabia. Asian Pac J Trop Dis. 2014; 4(1): 14-17.

[30] Malik A, Saxena NC. Ultrasound in abdominal tuberculosis. Abdom Imaging. 2003; 28(4): 574-579.

[31] Reed DH, Nash AF, Valabhji P. Radiological diagnosis and management of a solitary tubercular hepatic abscess. Br J Surg. 1990; 63: 902-904.

[32] Chan SG, Pang J. Isolated giant tuberculomata of the liver detected by computed tomography. Gastrointest Radiol. 1989; 14: 305-307.

[33] Tirumani SH, Ojili V, Gunabushanam G, Shanbhogue AKP, Nagar A, Fasih N, et al. Imaging of tuberculosis of the abdominal viscera: beyond the intestines. J Clin Imaging Sci. 2013; 3(1): 17.

[34] Chatterjee S, Schmid ML, Anderson K, Oppong KW. Tuberculosis and the pancreas: a diagnostic challenge solved by endoscopic ultrasound. A case series. J Gastrointestin Liver Dis. 2012; 21(1): 105-107.

[35] Rana SS, Sharma V, Sharma R, Bhasin DK. Involvement of mediastinal/intra-abdominal lymph nodes, spleen, liver, and left adrenal in presumed isolated pancreatic tuberculosis: an endoscopic ultrasound study. J Digest Endosc. 2015; 6 (1): 15.

[36] Diehl DL, Johal AS, Shieh FK, Ramesh J, Varadarajulu S, Ali A, et al. Su 1583 endoscopic ultrasound-guided liver biopsy: a multicenter experience. Gastrointest Endosc. 2013; 77(5): 375.

[37] Uzunkoy A, Harma M. Diagnosis of abdominal tuberculosis: experience from 11 cases and review of the literature. World J Gastroenterol: WJG. 2004; 10(24): 3647-3649.

[38] Tuberculosis. NICE guidelines [NG33] 2016.

[39] Samant H, Desai D, Abraham P, Joshi A, Gupta T, Rodrigues C, et al. Acid-fast bacilli culture positivity and drug resistance in abdominal tuberculosis in Mumbai, India. Indian J Gastroenterol. 2014; 33(5): 414-419.

[40] Lee JY. Diagnosis and treatment of extrapulmonary tuberculosis. Tuberc Respir Dis. 2015; 78(2): 47-55.

[41] Reynolds TB, Campra JL, Peters RL. Hepatic granulomata. In: Zakim D, Boyer TD, editors. Hepatology — a textbook of liver disease. 2nd ed. Philadelphia: WB

Saunders; 1990. p. 1098.
[42] Alvarez SZ. Hepatobiliary tuberculosis. Phil J Gastroenterol. 2006; 2: 1-10.
[43] Korn RJ, Kellow WF, Heller P, et al. Hepatic involvement in extrapulmonary tuberculosis: histologic and functional characteristics. Am J Med. 1959; 27: 60-71.
[44] Ramesh J, Banait GS, Ormerod LP. Abdominal tuberculosis in a district general hospital: a retrospective review of 86 cases. Q J Med. 2008; 101(3): 189-195.
[45] King TC, Upfal M, Gottlieb A, Adamo P, Bernacki E, Kadlecek CP, et al. T-SPOT. TB interferon-γ release assay performance in healthcare worker screening at nineteen US hospitals. Am J Respir Crit Care Med. 2015; 192(3): 367-373.
[46] World Health O. Implementing tuberculosis diagnostics: policy. Framework. 2015.
[47] Saukkonen JJ, Cohn DL, Jasmer RM, et al. An official ATS statement: hepatotoxicity of antituberculous therapy. Am J Respir Crit Care Med. 2006; 174: 935-952.
[48] Xing X, Li H, Liu WG. Hepatic segmentectomy for treatment of hepatic tuberculous pseudotumor. Hepatobiliary Pancreat Dis Int. 2005; 4: 565-568.
[49] Thomas MR, Goldin RD. Tuberculosis presenting as jaundice. Brit J Clin Pract. 1990; 44: 161-163.
[50] Mandak M, Kerbl U, Kleinert R, et al. Miliare tuberkulose der lebere als ursache eines septischen schocks mit multiorganversagen as this seems to be a rather long word. Wien Klin Wschr. 1999; 106: 111-114.

脾结核

[51] Meredith HC, Early JQ, Becker W. Tuberculous splenomegaly with the hypersplenism syndrome. Blood. 1949; 4: 1367-1373.
[52] Lin SF, Zheng L, Zhou L. Solitary splenic tuberculosis: a case report and review of the literatüre. World J Surg Oncol. 2016; 14: 154.
[53] Basa JV, Singh L, Jaoude WA, Sugiyama G. A case of isolated splenic tuberculosis. Int J Surg Case Rep. 2015; 8: 117-119.
[54] Imani Fooladi AA, Hosseini MJ, Azizi T. Splenic tuberculosis: a case report. Int J Infect Dis. 2009; 13(5): e273-275.
[55] Raviraj S, Gogia A, Kakar A, Byotra SP. Isolated splenic tuberculosis without any radiological focal lesion. Case Rep Med. 2015; 2015: 2.
[56] Kumar A, Kapoor VK, Behari A, Verma S. Splenic tuberculosis in a immunocompetent patient can be managed conservatively: a case report. Gastroenterol Rep. 2015: 1-3.
[57] Nasa M, Choudhary NS, Gulerşa M, Puri R. Isolated splenic tuberculosis diagnosed by endoscopic ultrasound-guided fine needle aspiration. Indian J Tuberc. 2017; 64(2): 134-135.
[58] Azzam NA. Splenic tuberculosis presenting as fever of unknown origin with severe neutropenia. Ann Clin Microbiol Antimicrob. 2013; 12(1): 1-3.
[59] Gupta PP, Fotedar S, Agarwal D, Sansanwal P. Tuberculosis of spleen presenting with pyrexia of unknown origin in a non-immunocompromised woman. Lung India. 2008; 25(1): 22-24.

[60] Mishra H, Pradeep R, Rao GV, Anuradha S, Reddy DN. Isolated tuberculosis of the spleen: a case report and review of literature. Indian J Surg. 2013; 75(3): 235-236.
[61] Jain D, Verma K, Jain P. Disseminated tuberculosis causing isolated splenic vein thrombosis and multiple splenic abscesses. Oxf Med Case Rep. 2014; (6): 107-109.
[62] Harries A, Maher D. TB: A Clinical Manual for South-East Asia. Geneva: World Health Organisation; 1997. p. 32-33.
[63] Tiri B, Saraca LM, Luciano E, Burkert FR, Cappanera S, Cenci E, Francisci D. Splenic tuberculosis in a patient with newly diagnosed advanced HIV infection. IDCases. 2016; 6: 20-22.
[64] Montales MT, Caudhury A, Beebe A, Patil S, Patil N. HIV-associated TB syndemic: a growing clinical challenge. Front Public Health. 2015; 3: 281.
[65] Sotgiu G, Migliori GB. Extra-pulmonary tuberculosis: the comorbidity of the near future? Int J Tuberc Lung Dis. 2014; 18(12): 1389.
[66] Hamizah R, Rohana AG, Anwar SA, Ong TZ, Hamazaini AH, Zuikarnaen AN. Splenic tuberculosis presenting as pyrexia of unknown origin. Med J Malaysia. 2007; 62(1): 70-71.
[67] Pottakkat B, Kumar A, Rastogi A, Krishnani N, Kapoor VK, Saxena R. Tuberculosis of the spleen as a cause of fever of unknown origin and splenomegaly. Gut Liver. 2010; 4(1): 94-97.
[68] Zaleznik DF, Kasper DL. Intra-abdominal infections and abscesses. In: Fauci AS, Braunwald Isselbacher KJ, et al., editors. Harrison's principles of internal medicine, vol. 1. 14th ed. New York: McGraw Hill Company; 1998. p. 792-796.
[69] World Health Organization. Global tuberculosis report; 2016.
[70] Wangai F, Achieng L, Otieno G, Njoroge J, Wambaire T, Rajab J. Isolated splenic tuberculosis with subsequent paradoxical deterioration: a case report. BMC Res Notes. 2017; 10: 162.
[71] Yan D, Zhong CL, Li LJ. Systemic spread of tuberculosis after surgery for a splenic tuberculous abscess without postoperational antituberculosis treatment: a case report. Ther Clin Risk Manag. 2015; 11: 1697-1700.
[72] Lee KJ, Yoo JS, Jeon H, Cho SK, Lee JH, Ha SS, Cho MY, Kim JW. A case of splenic tuberculosis forming a gastro-splenic fistula. Korean J Gastroenterol. 2015; 66(3): 168-171.
[73] Zhan F, Wang C-J, Lin J-Z, Zhong P-J, Qiu W-Z, Lin H-H, et al. Isolated splenic tuberculosis: a case report. World J Gastrointest Pathophysiol. 2010; 1 (3): 109-111.
[74] Ho PL, Chim CS, Yuen KY. Isolated splenic tuberculosis presenting with pyrexia of unknown origin. Scand J Infect Dis. 2000; 32(6): 700-701.
[75] Bastounis E, Pikoulis E, Varelas P, Cirochristos D, Aessopos A. Tuberculoma of the spleen: a rare but important clinical entity. Am Surg. 1999; 65(2): 131-132.
[76] Mazloom W, Marion A, Ferron C, Lucht F, Mosnier JF. Tuberculose splenique: a partir d'un cas et revue de la literature. Medecine et Maladies Infectieuse. 2002; 32: 444-446.
[77] Rhazal F, Lahlou MK, Benamer S, Daghri JM, Essadel E, Mohammadine E,

et al. Splenomegalie et pseudotumeur splenique d'origine tuberculeuse: six nouvelles observations. Ann Chir. 2004; 129: 410-414.
[78] Berady S, Rabhi M, Bahrouch L, Sair K, Benziane H, Benkirane A, et al. Isolated pseudo-tumoral tuberculosis of the spleen. A case report. La revue de medecine interne/fondee par la Societe nationale francaise de. medecine interne. 2005; 26(7): 588-591.
[79] Cobelschi C, Maier A, Hogea MD, Gheorghiu AR, Toader I. Splenic tuberculosis — case report. Chirurgia (Bucur). 2016; 111(2): 165-169.
[80] Ortega S, Vizcairo A, Aguirre IB, et al. Tuberculosis as risk factor for venous thrombosis. An Med Intern. 1993; 10: 398-400.
[81] Zhang Y, Zhang J, Chen T, Zeng H, Zhao B, Zhang Y, Zhou X, Han W, Hu Y, Liu F, Shan Z, Gao W, Zhou H. Spontaneous splenic rupture in an acute leukemia patient with splenic tuberculosis a case report. Mol Clin Oncol. 2017; 6(2): 209-213.
[82] Sharma SK, Smith-Rohrberg D, Tahir M, Mohan A, Seith A. Radiological manifestations of splenic tuberculosis: a 23-patient case series from India. Indian J Med Res. 2007; 125: 669-678.
[83] Confer BD, Hanouneh I, Gomes M, Alraies MC. Is anticoagulation appropriate for all portal vein thrombosis? Cleve Clin J Med. 2013; 80: 612-613.

5
淋巴结结核

雅库普·哈坎·巴沙兰

5.1 流行病学

以前,在希波克拉底时代,"瘰疬"被用来指代所有的颈部淋巴结肿胀。自1882年结核杆菌被发现后,导致淋巴结疾病因素被区分开来,由结核分枝杆菌引起疾病被命名为腺结核病。此外,还明确了结核分枝杆菌不是导致淋巴结疾病的唯一因素。

结核杆菌引起的淋巴结炎主要见于儿童,被认为是儿童肺结核的表现。米勒·乔治·P(Müller George P)公布了一份最早的关于结核性淋巴结炎的统计学报告,报告指出结核性淋巴结炎发病率最高的年龄段是2~17岁。到20世纪70年代,随着防治措施的完善和提高,结核病的总体发病率下降。威廉·C.沃尔桑格(William C Voorsanger)在1937年说明了结核病的病死率从325/100万人下降到58/100万人,主要下降群体在1~10岁年龄段,通常是淋巴结结核患者。特别是自20世纪70年代以来,随着HIV病毒感染的迅速蔓延,淋巴结结核的平均发病间隔从儿童时期改为20~40岁。另外血液恶性肿瘤疾病的增加和为了预防器官移植中的排斥反应使用免疫抑制剂,也导致了成人结核病及其并发症的上升。伊尔加兹利(Ilgazli)等人在一项研究中搜集了从1岁到89岁的636例病例,发现肺外结核病例的平均年龄为22.5岁。米哈伊·鲁阿尔·波佩斯库(Mihai Raul Popescu)进行的另一项研究包含了362个EPTB的案例,结果显示平均年龄为35岁。来自埃塞俄比亚西北部的穆鲁耶(Muluye)等人公布了淋巴结结核患病率最高的年龄组是15~24岁,其次是25~34岁。

结核分枝杆菌复合体是由微生物组成的群体,是导致淋巴结结核的主要原因。其中包含了人结核分枝杆菌、牛分枝杆菌、非洲分枝杆菌、微小分枝杆菌、犬分支枝杆菌。分枝杆菌的主要目标是肺,但杆菌可能在活动期或潜伏再激活期间从肺向其他器官和组织扩散并形成肺外结核,淋巴结结核是肺外结核最常见的表现形式。此外,当未经过巴氏消毒的污染奶制品被消费时,牛结核分枝杆菌和各种非结核分枝杆菌可能导致尤其是颈部淋巴结的感染。

美国疾病预防控制中心在 2016 年结核病监测报告中指出,在整个美国肺结核、肺外结核、同时患有肺结核和肺外结核的病例,分别增加了 69.6%、20.3%和 9.9%。报告还指出,在所有受分枝杆菌影响的肺外组织中,淋巴组织是结核最常见的肺外目标,其占比高达 35.8%。结核性淋巴结炎可能感染所有的淋巴组织,但最常见的感染区域是颈部淋巴区。

从统计数据上来看,肺外结核除了对共患疾病,还对跨地域感染造成很大影响。据报道,在结核高负荷的国家,肺外结核发病率更高。世卫组织2017 年全球结核病报告显示全球和世卫组织非洲区域、美洲区域、东地中海区域、欧洲区域、东南亚区域、西太平洋区域的肺外结核发病率百分比分别为 15%、16%、15%、24%、15%、15%和 8%。欧洲疾病预防控制中心 2013 年的报告公布了全欧盟的肺外结核病例占比为 22.3%,同时期美国报告公布了全美肺外结核病例占比为 30.2%。另外一作者特雷莎·戈马斯 (Teresa Gomes)等人报道了 2007 年至 2011 年,巴西的肺外结核病例总数占比为 17%。

性别和出生地在淋巴结结核的发展中也起着重要的作用。虽然结核病在男性中更常见,但是肺外结核却在女性中更常见。统计报告通常显示男女比例为 1∶1.4。在罗马尼亚的一项包括大量病例的研究中,米哈伊·鲁阿尔·波佩斯库报告了男性/女性淋巴结结核病例的比率为 0.63。此外,波佩斯库表示尽管患有淋巴结结核合并其他部位感染的患者多为男性,但是单纯患有淋巴结结核的患者多为女性。

生活在结核高负荷或低负荷地区和社会经济条件不仅影响结核病和肺外结核,还影响了淋巴结结核发病率。T. 高·布朗(T. Gow Brown)讨论了生活在不健康环境中的影响并指出在不健康条件下结核病的所有表现都会增加。不利的环境和弱势的地位也使淋巴结结核发生的高峰移向儿童时期。

免疫抑制条件的共存显著增加了结核病的所有肺外表现,例如淋巴结结核。在巴西的一项研究中,特雷莎·戈马斯发现 EPTB 病例与没有并发症的肺结核病例相比几乎翻了一倍。

由宁·C(Naing C)等人进行的 meta 分析，表明 HIV 与 EPTB 之间存在显著的联系。HIV 相关的免疫抑制影响了结核病的临床表现，同时也增加了肺外结核的发病率。53%～63%的 HIV 患者有单独发生 EPTB 的倾向。

5.2 发病机制

结核分枝杆菌主要目标是肺部，但传播其他器官的情况并不罕见。淋巴组织是结核分枝杆菌最常见的肺外目标。感染淋巴结的结核杆菌可能是通过接触开放的伤口或通过消化道进入体内成为主要传染源，再经淋巴管或血源性传播的方法传播到组织中。

当结核杆菌越过上呼吸道的初级防御系统进入肺泡，随即被肺泡巨噬细胞所吞噬。通常大多数细菌在被巨噬细胞吞噬后，会被巨噬细胞内富含裂解酶的溶酶体和吞噬体融合而消灭，但结核分枝杆菌被吞噬后并没有被吞噬体和溶酶体融合而消灭，而是通过它的各种表面分子与初级防御系统相互作用，在吞噬体或细胞质中增殖，直到离开巨噬细胞。研究表明，在结核杆菌到达淋巴结后细胞免疫开始启动，抗原特异性 T 细胞被激活发挥出抗结核作用，树突状细胞在这过程中起着重要作用。

另一方面，结核分枝杆菌是一种生长缓慢的微生物。树突细胞将细菌呈递到淋巴结，直到细菌达到足够的数量才能被识别和呈现。接着，当细菌出现在淋巴结时，效应 T 淋巴细胞开始分化，这些效应 T 淋巴细胞向感染区域迁移发挥出细胞防御的作用。因此，淋巴结是肺外结核感染最常见的部位并不奇怪。

此外，从呼吸道进入的结核杆菌并不总是能到达淋巴结。另一种分枝杆菌，牛分枝杆菌，可能被口服摄入，引起尤其是颈部和腹部淋巴结炎。一些国家的动物被牛分枝杆菌感染，并且在消费它们的奶时未经巴氏消毒，导致牛分枝杆菌引起的颈部淋巴结炎在这些国家中占了很大比例。

5.3 临床表现

由于结核分枝杆菌的亚型不同，淋巴结核影响的淋巴结根据频率排列依次为颈锁骨上、纵隔、腋窝和腹股沟淋巴结。颈部淋巴结受累的百分比在63%~77%。因此临床描述和症状学的研究主要围绕的是颈部淋巴结结核。大部分患者的主诉为在颈后或锁骨上发现无痛、缓慢长大的淋巴结。因此,当患者出现淋巴结增生,并且抗生素治疗无效,尤其是来自疫区,必须进行评估是否是淋巴结结核。

马德格达拉(Madegedara)等人在斯里兰卡一个疫区的研究中,分析了152例孤立肺外结核患者受淋巴结影响的频率,结果见下表(表5-1)。

表5-1 152例孤立肺外结核患者受淋巴结影响的频率

影 响 部 位	百 分 比(%)
颈 部	78.94
腋 窝	11.18
颈部和腋窝	3.28
颌 下	3.28
锁骨上	1.31
腹股沟	1.31
腹股沟和腋窝	0.66

淋巴结结核全身症状包括低热、易疲劳和体重减轻。然而,幼儿和免疫功能低下的HIV阳性患者可能会出现明显的发热症状和淋巴结迅速扩大。

增生是受感染的淋巴组织最先出现的反应,通常在感染的数周或数月内发生。逐渐形成肉芽肿。淋巴结最初是坚实、可移动、孤立地附着在周围组织上。大约10%的病例可能发生肿大的淋巴结引流。通常该区域波及一个以上的淋巴结,其中一个淋巴结突出并且不对称地增大。受累的淋巴结逐渐发生干酪样坏死。由于坏死,受累的淋巴结产生液体内容物并有波动感。随后,淋巴结的内容物可能通过形成的瘘管自由排出。这种排液可能持续几个月。

尽管给予足够的药物治疗,肿胀的淋巴结可能抵抗并形成"冷脓肿"。还可以与其他细菌共同感染引起周围性淋巴炎伴有其他炎症迹象,例如发热、变色、疼痛。患有肺结核同时伴有淋巴结结核的患者主诉通常包括经典的肺结核症状,咳血、胸痛、体重下降、疲劳、发热、盗汗和寒战。伴随有HIV和儿童患儿也会出现典型的结核病症状。

由波佩斯库(Popescu)等人进行的回顾性研究证实了几乎所有的患者

都不是单个淋巴结受累而是整个淋巴结群受累。此外,在同一研究中,可以得出结论,单个淋巴结粘连比多个被感染的淋巴结更常见。到目前为止,在淋巴结结核里,多发性淋巴结受累以淋巴结增大和干酪样坏死为主要临床表现。由于颈部淋巴结是淋巴结结核最常见的一组淋巴结群,观察淋巴结的临床变化更容易。为了从临床上辨别淋巴结结核,琼斯(Jones)和坎伯尔(Campbell)在1962年对淋巴结结核进行5个阶段分类将有助于识别该疾病。

(1) 第1期,淋巴结肿大、坚实、可移动、孤立,表现为非特异性增生;

(2) 第2期,由于周围炎症,肿大的橡胶样的淋巴结被固定在周围组织上;

(3) 第3期,脓肿形成导致中央软化;

(4) 第4期,领扣样脓肿形成;

(5) 第5期,窦道形成。

临床上,从解剖可见位置发现淋巴结结核是容易的,但怀疑其他部位的淋巴结结核是更困难的。这些病例的临床症状取决于区域淋巴引流的堵塞和对周围组织结构的压迫效应。

纵隔淋巴结结核:咳嗽和胸痛可能是纵隔疾病的主要症状。然而,邻近组织的压迫也可能成为淋巴结肿大的征象。当淋巴结压迫一个肺,患者可能出现肺不张或体位性呼吸困难,食管压迫引起吞咽困难或心脏压塞,导致食管穿孔和食管气管瘘形成也有报道。

腋下淋巴结结核:如果没有肺结核存在,可能会发展为无痛、逐渐扩大腋窝肿块。可能导致淋巴引流阻塞和腋前组织肿胀。

腹膜淋巴结结核:经常累及门静脉周围、胰周和肠系膜淋巴结。Baik SJ等人报道一例胆总管周围淋巴结结核引起的梗阻性黄疸。

5.4 诊断

大多数情况下当结核病灶出现在一个可见的区域很容易被疑似是结核病。然而,要做到正确的诊断仍然具有一定困难。在结核病流行区,淋巴结结核患者应该仔细询问与结核病患者的接触情况、以前的结核病病史、生活环境、典型症状、伴随疾病,尤其是HIV、出汗时间以及淋巴结肿大的特征变化。有了怀疑,实验室检查也是必不可少的。然而,没有任何实验室检测肯定不能百分之百排除结核病。

1. Mantoux试验(结核菌素皮肤试验)：Mantoux试验在诊断结核性疾病，特别是潜在结核病例中仍然是一项有价值的试验。测试的初始步骤是将5个结核菌素单位(TU)(0.1 ml)的纯化蛋白衍生物用皮内注射的方法注入前臂一个无毛发的区域，并在48～72 h后测量硬结的大小。该试验的不利方面包括需要对患者复诊检查，以及由于患者之前接种疫苗而产生难以解释结果。虽然它在应用上有困难，但拉基·M(Lakhey M)强调了Mantoux试验，一项由122例淋巴结核病例组成的研究，认为细胞学、染色和Mantoux试验的结合提高了诊断淋巴结结核的效率。

2. 抗酸染色，Erlich-Ziehl-Neelsen染色(EZN)：当同时伴有活动性肺结核时，使用经典的抗酸染色(acid-fast staining, AFS)方法有更高的概率来识别细菌，但是，为了成功的明确细菌种类需要高载量的细菌样本，大约每毫升需要超过1 000个细菌才能明确。尽管细菌的载量对EZN的阳性结果很重要，但肺标本的总体灵敏度为71.4%，肺外标本为24%。此外，从引流瘘管中搜集的或从淋巴结取得的具有检查价值的其他临床样本，尽管结果仍有假阳性和假阴性可能，但EZN结果的阳性高度明确了结核杆菌的感染。

3. 组织病理学检查：对受累淋巴结标本的组织病理学检查给出了高度特异性的结果。受累淋巴结标本可以通过几种方式收集。首先细针抽吸(fine needle aspiration, FNA)具有较少的侵入性和较容易的特点。根据受影响淋巴结的位置，抽吸可以用一个简单的注射器或使用复杂的技术进行，如支气管镜或胃镜。在一些临床情况下，如一个固定和坚硬的肿块，这是不可能抽吸的，切除活检是完整取出肿大淋巴结的办法。该方法获得的标本可用于EZN染色、细菌培养、快速检测和组织病理学检查。淋巴样浸润，非干酪样肉芽肿和肉芽肿内干酪样改变与朗格汉斯巨细胞增生是淋巴结核的组织学指标。虽然FNA比切除活检的侵入性小，但各种研究的结论是切除活检对淋巴结结核的确诊有更大的价值。

4. 细菌培养：培养基上结核杆菌生长是诊断结核病的金标准。然而，结核杆菌在培养基里的生长是缓慢的(通常需要2～4周)，同时培养的阴性结果不能排除这种疾病。从受累的淋巴结中获得的标本，特别是切除活检的，具有最高的诊断价值。痰或血培养对结核病诊断可能也有帮助。

5. 聚合酶链反应(polymerase chain reaction, PCR)：在发达国家和发展中国家广泛应用。Aljaferi等人2004年发表了一项研究，结论是PCR作为一种更快速、更可靠的检测方法,可以快速地定性来自研究中的96.2%的结核分枝杆菌感染病例。

6. 核酸扩增试验(nucleic acid amplification tests, NAATs):有商业上可用的NAATs;结核分枝杆菌扩增直接试验(MTD, Gen-Probe)、XpertMTB/RIF(通常称为GeneXpert)、焦磷酸测序和自制。

(1) Gen-Probe MTD试验是FDA为抗酸杆菌(acid-fast bacilli, AFB)阳性患者宣布和批准的第一个NAAT。1999年后期,增强MTD(E-MTD)也被批准用于AFB阴性患者。测试的原理是转录介导的扩增和靶向结核分枝杆菌核糖体RNA。其敏感性超过70%,AFB阳性病例显著增加。测试的特异性是98%。

(2) 在2013年,XpertMTB/RIF被FDA批准用于检测所有类型的临床标本中的结核分枝杆菌。该试验在高负担国家具有较高的敏感性,也用于检测利福平的耐药性。Chang等人以药敏试验和培养物为金标准进行meta分析,并将试验的敏感性和特异性公布分别为95%和98%。测试的其他优点包括基于自动检测盒、无污染和快速得到结果。结果可在2h以内得到。

(3) 焦磷酸测序(pyrosequencing, PSQ)也是另一种核酸扩增试验,通常负责检测耐药的突变。PSQ可用于AFB阳性标本和利福平、异烟肼和喹诺酮的耐药突变检测。

(4) HAIN是一种尚未得到FDA批准的检测异烟肼、利福平和喹诺酮类耐药的线探针检测方法。

7. 影像学检查:根据受累淋巴结的定位,成像技术可能可以作为替代方式。

(1) 胸部X线片是结核病的首选成像技术。它易于做到、廉价并且能成功地显示钙化;因此,它仍然是一个用于诊断肺结核的首选检查,但超声检查对于淋巴结结核更方便。

(2) 超声检查:由于主要定位于颈部淋巴结,超声检查有利于确定受累淋巴结的数量、形状和质地、粘连、测量淋巴结的大小和探索是否有邻近的软组织水肿。周围软组织水肿、淋巴结内坏死、粘连和后续治疗改进是评价淋巴结结核对抗转移性淋巴结增大的有用的标准。随着坏死的发展,淋巴结的同质结构改变,中心可被视为一个异质性区域。此外,超声可能有助于引导从淋巴结中进行针刺抽吸(FNA)。

（3）CT和MRI对于诊断淋巴结结核是有价值的。用三维模型显示受累淋巴结的解剖结构以及受累淋巴结与邻近组织的关系,在CT上以低信号、在MRI的T2像上以高信号显示中央坏死区是该检查对于诊断有利的一面。此外,CT是评估腹部淋巴结结核的最佳选择,但用这些方法鉴别结核坏死和鳞状细胞癌仍有困难。由于放射性高,CT将不是显示淋巴结的首选检查;此外,为了看到钙化中心,将需要使用静脉造影剂,这对患者来说可能是有毒的。MRI可以在这些条件下替代CT,但MRI很贵,而且在许多设施中都没有。

（4）PET-CT是一种常用于检查肿瘤转移的方法。昂贵、耗时,在大多数设施中几乎没有。对淋巴结结核的诊断研究价值仍有争议。然而,它可能有助于区分肺结核的一些形式,如肺和淋巴形式。此外,一些研究人员报告了PET-CT有助于跟踪抗结核治疗的反应。

8. 实验室检查

（1）红细胞沉降率(ESR)通常升高,但对淋巴结结核并不特异。

（2）IFN-γ释放试验(IGRAs):结核分枝杆菌不同于大多数其他环境分枝杆菌和减毒结核分枝杆菌(又称为卡介苗,用于世界各地的结核病疫苗接种)。基因组中的差异称为"差异区域"(RD1)。RD1区域编码9种蛋白质。该方法的主要原则是在疑似患者中确定RD1的存在。结核分枝杆菌感染者的白细胞与抗原结合后会释放IFN-γ。在临床上RD1存在提示结核分枝杆菌感染,在接种卡介苗或受环境分枝杆菌感染的患者中该试验呈阴性。经FDA批准的两种IGRA是QuantiFERON-TB Gold In-Tube(QFT-GIT)试验和T-SPOT结核试验(T-Spot)。

a. QuantiFERON-TB Gold In-Tube试验:ESAT-6、CFP-10和TB7.7是作为结核分枝杆菌抗原的三种合成肽,是一种单独的混合物。使用该方法测定IFN-γ浓度。

b. T-SPOT结核试验:两种蛋白质,即RD1的ESAT-6和CFP-10,用于激活患者的T细胞。识别这两种蛋白质的效应T细胞开始释放IFN-γ。

当天得到结果和不需要复诊是IGRA的优点。然而,高成本和所需的复杂技术使低收入国家的测试不太可行。因此,WHO不但建议IGRAs取代Mantoux试验,还建议在低收入国家IGRAs用于活动性结核病的诊断。疾病预防控制中心建议在特殊条件下,如作为对接触者、孕妇和保健工作者筛查而使用这些测试方法。

5.5 鉴别诊断

虽然绝大多数淋巴结肿大，特别是在高负荷国家，淋巴结结核是病因，但其他几个病因必须记住，例如其他感染淋巴结的原因（如弓形虫病、巴尔通体病、真菌感染、土拉菌病）、原发性淋巴结恶性肿瘤（尤其是淋巴瘤）和转移灶、自身免疫性疾病、药物反应以及其他一些综合征像结节病、囊性纤维化和储存障碍作为鉴别诊断必须记住。一般的诊断方法是从良好的病史、良好的检查、FNA 细胞学检查和 GeneXpert 测试开始，以鉴别淋巴结结核。

5.6 治疗

确定淋巴结炎的致病因素和耐药性对治疗的选择至关重要。IDSA 建议无耐药性结核分枝杆菌引起的淋巴结结核治疗为异烟肼、利福平、吡嗪酰胺、乙胺丁醇 2 个月，异烟肼和利福平 4 个月。

在治疗过程中，可能会出现矛盾的淋巴结增大、新的淋巴结受累和新的引流窦形成。矛盾反应可能发生在 20%～23% 的 HIV 血清阴性患者。在 HIV 阳性患者中，由于使用抗逆转录病毒疗法，明确使矛盾反应更为复杂。

手术作为非结核性淋巴结炎的首选，治愈率超过 70%。此外，手术切除可应用在治疗过程中出现矛盾反应的患者、不符合治疗的患者和对现有淋巴结增大或引流淋巴结感到不舒服的患者。然而即使做了手术，也是建议使用抗生素的。

5.7 后续观察

积极的治疗标准是改善临床症状和缩小淋巴结的大小。此外，如果需要，GeneXpert 试验有助于跟踪治疗反应。

参考文献

[1] Aaron L. Tuberculosis in HIV-infected patients: a comprehensive review. CMI. 2004; 10(5): 388-398.

[2] Aljaferi AS. Diagnosis of tuberculous lymphadenitis by FNAC, microbiological methods and PCR: a comparative study. Cytopathology. 2004; 15(1): 44-48.
[3] Baik SJ. A case of obstructive jaundice caused by tuberculous lymphadenitis: A literature review. Clin Mol Hepatol. 2014; 20(2): 208-213.
[4] Bem C. Human Immunodeficiency virus positive tuberculosis lymphadenitis in central africa: clinical presentation of 157 cases. Int J Tuberc Lung Dis. 1995; 20: 876-882.
[5] Brown TG. The influence of social factors on the incidence of extra-pulmonary tuberculosis infection. J Hyg (Lond). 1947; 45(2): 239-250.
[6] Tuberculosis-United States, 2016. MMWR 2017; 66(11); 289-294.
[7] Chackerian A, Alt J, Perera T, Dascher C. SMB Dissemination of Mycobacterium tuberculosis is influenced by host factors and precedes the initiation of T-cell immunity. Infect Immun. 2002; 70: 4501-4509.
[8] Chandir S. Extrapulmonary tuberculosis: a retrospective review of 194 cases at a tertiary care hospital in Karachi, Pakistan. J Pak Med Assoc. 2010; 60(2): 105-109.
[9] Chang K, et al. Rapid and effective diagnosis of tuberculosis and rifampin resistance with Xpert MTB/RIF assay: a meta-analysis. J Infect. 2012; 64(6): 580-588.
[10] Cho OH, Park KH, Kim T, et al. Paradoxical responses in non-HIV-infected patients with peripheral lymph node tuberculosis. J Infect. 2009; 59: 56-61.
[11] Demangel C, Bertolino P, Britton WJ. Autocrine IL-10 impairs dendritic cell (DC)-derived immune responses to mycobacterial infection by suppressing DC trafficking to draining lymph nodes and local IL-12 production. Eur J Immunol. 2002; 32: 994-1002.
[12] European Centre for Disease Prevention and Cotrol Annual epidemiological report Reporting on 2011 surveillance data and 2012 epidemic intelligence data. 2013.
[13] Geldmacher H. Assessment of lymph node tuberculosis in northern Germany: a clinical review. Chest. 2002; 121(4): 1177-1182.
[14] Gomes T. Epidemiology of extrapulmonary tuberculosis in Brazil: a hierarchical model. BMC Infect Dis. 2014; 14: 9.
[15] Hatipoğlu N and Güvenç H. (2017). Chapter 4 Peripheral Tuberculous Lymphadenitis: Clinical Approach and Medico-Surgical Management.
[16] Hawkey CR, Yap T, Pereira J, et al. Characterization and management of paradoxical upgrading reactions in HIV-uninfected patients with lymph node tuberculosis. Clin Infect Dis. 2005; 40: 1368-1371.
[17] Ilgazlı A. Extrapulmonary tuberculosis: clinical and epidemiologic spectrum of 636 cases. Arch Med Res. 2004; 35(5): 435-441.
[18] Kanlıkama M. Management strategy of mycobacterial cervical lymphadenitis. J Laryngol Otol. 2000; 114: 274-278.
[19] Karadağ A. Comparison of culture, real-time DNA amplification assay and erlich-ziehl-neelsen for detection of mycobacterium tuberculosis. Balkan Med J. 2013; 30 (1): 13-15.
[20] Khader S, Partida-Sanchez S, Bell G, Jelley-Gibbs D, Swain S, et al. Interleukin

12p40 is required for dendritic cell migration and T cell priming after Mycobacterium tuberculosis infection. J Exp Med. 2006; 203: 1805-1815.

[21] Lakhey M. Diagnosis of tubercular lymphadenopathy by fine needle aspiration cytology, acid-fast staining and Mantoux test. JNMA J Nepal Med Assoc. 2009; 48(175): 230-233.

[22] Lee KC. Contemporary management of cervical tuberculosis. Laryngoscope. 1992; 102(1): 60-64.

[23] Mert A. Tuberculous lymphadenopathy in adults: a review of 35 cases. Acta Chir Belg. 2002; 102(2): 118-121.

[24] Müller GP. The Treatment of Tuberculous Cervical Lymphadenitis. Annals of Surgery 1913; LVIII(4): 433-450.

[25] Muluye D. Prevalence of tuberculous lymphadenitis in Gondar University Hospital, Northwest Ethiopia. BMC Public Health. 2013; 13: 435.

[26] Naing C. Meta-analysis: the association between HIV infection and extrapulmonary tuberculosis. Lung. 2013; 191(1): 27-34.

[27] Okten I, Management of esophageal perforation. Surg Today. 2001; 31(1): 36-39.

[28] Panesar J, Higgins K, Daya H, Forte V, Allen U. Nontuberculous mycobacterial cervical adenitis: a ten-year retrospective review. Laryngoscope. 2003; 113: 149-154.

[29] Paredes C, Delcampo F, Zamarron C, et al. Cardiac tamponade due to tuberculous mediastinal lymphadenitis. Tubercle. 1990; 71: 219-220.

[30] Perlman DC, D'Amico R, Salomon N. Mycobacterial diseases of the head and the neck. Curr Inf Dis Rep. 2001; 3(3): 233.

[31] Polesky A. Peripheral tuberculous lymphadenitis: epidemiology, diagnosis, treatment, and outcome. Medicine. 2005; 84(6): 350-362.

[32] Raul M. Popescu Lymph Node Tuberculosis- an attempt of clinico-morphological study and review of the literature. Rom J Morphol Embryol. 2014; 55: 553-567.

[33] Rodriguez et al. Enfermedades infecciosas y microbiologia clinica vol 29 num 7 agosto settembre. 2011; 29: 502-509.

[34] Shafer RW. Extrapulmonary tuberculosis in patients with human immunodeficiency virus infection. Medicine (Baltimore). 1991; 70: 384-397.

[35] Singh KK. Comparison of in-house polymerase chain reaction with conventional techniques for the detection of Mycobacterium tuberculosis DNA in granulomatous lymphadenopathy. J Clin Pathol. 2000; 53(5): 355-361.

[36] Singh B, Moodly M, Goga AD, Haffejee AA, et al. Dysphagia secondary to tuberculous lymphadenitis. S Afr J Surg. 1996; 34: 197-199.

[37] Soussan M, Brillet PY, Mekinian A, Khafagy A, Nicolas P, Vessieres A, Brauner M. Patterns of pulmonary tuberculosis on FDG-PET/CT. Eur J Radiol. 2012; 81: 2872-2876.

[38] Spyridis P. Mycobacterial cervical Lymphadenitis in children: clinical and laboratory factors of importance for differential diagnosis. Scand J Infect Dis. 2001; 33(5).

[39] Tan CH, Kontoyiannis DP, Viswanathan C, Iyer RB. Tuberculosis: a benign impostor. Am J Roentengenol. 2010; 194: 555-561.

[40] Tian G, Xiao Y, Chen B, Xia J, Guan H, Deng Q. FDG PET/CT for therapeutic

response monitoring in multi-site non-respiratory tuberculosis. Acta Radiol. 2010; 51: 1002 - 1006.
[41] Centers for Disease Control and Preventation, Treatment of tuberculosis, MMWR Recomm Rep. 2003; 52: 1 - 77.
[42] William C. VORSANGER. Tuberculous Cervical Lymphadenitis. Cal West Med. 1937; 47(3): 194 - 198.
[43] World Health Organisation. Global Tuberculosis Report 2017.
[44] Wolf A, Desvignes L, Linas B, Banaiee N, Tamura T, et al. Initiation of the adaptive immune response to Mycobacterium tuberculosis depends on antigen production in the local lymph node, not the lungs. J Exp Med. 2008; 205: 105 - 115.
[45] Xiong L, et al. Posterior mediastinal lymphadenitis with dysphagia as the main symptom a case report and literature review. J Thorac Dis. 2013; 5(5): E189 - 194.
[46] Yadla M, Sivakumar V, Kalawat T. Assessment of early response to treatment in extrapulmonary tuberculosis: role of FDG-PET. Indian J Nucl Med. 2012; 27: 136 - 137.
[47] Ying M, Ahuja AT, Evans R, King W, Metreweli C. Cervical lymphadenopathy: sonographic differentiation between tuberculous nodes and nodal metastases from non-head and neck carcinomas. J Clin Ultrasound. 1998; 26: 383 - 389.
[48] Forssbohm M, Zwahlen M, Loddenkemper R, Rieder HL. Demographic characteristics of patients with extrapulmonary tuberculosis in Germany. European Respiratory Journal. 2008; 31(1): 99 - 105.
[49] Chan-Young. Extra-pulmonary and pulmonary tuberculosis in Hong Kong. Int J Tuberc Lung Dis. 2002; 6(10): 879 - 886.
[50] CDC. Trends in Tuberculosis — United States, 2008, MMWR March 20, 2009/ 58(10); 249 - 253.

6
结核性关节炎和结核性骨髓炎

居尔登·厄尔茨,奈菲斯·奥托普拉克和菲根·萨里德

6.1 结核性关节炎

6.1.1 流行病学

　　肌肉和骨结核是结核分枝杆菌导致的罕见的肺外并发症。骨关节结核在发展中国家仍然是一个常见的问题,所有在结核病流行率高的国家出生或居住的病例都应该考虑这个病。骨关节结核是一种继发型的结核病,最常见的原因是通过淋巴结逆行播散,而邻近播散是另一种不常见的传播方式,从一个原发的病灶,如肺、肾或淋巴结,或偶尔从邻近组织直接种植感染。约一半的病例脊柱受累,其余病例累及椎管外骨关节。骨关节结核占所有结核病例的1％～4.3％,占所有肺外结核病例的10％～15％,但由于免疫抑制患者和HIV感染人数的增加,这些病例的发病率一直在上升。罕见的是,腱鞘炎、滑囊炎或肌炎可能在较低发生率下发病。骨关节结核通常涉及身体的主干和负重关节。关节结核可能直接侵袭滑膜,如Poncet关节炎。此外,负重关节,如手腕、肘部和手的小关节也可能受累。关节疾病的结果是导致关节周围矿物质脱失,关节边缘部分侵蚀,支撑结构受损导致的滑膜炎。滑膜炎在关节损伤中迅速发生,尤其是在负重关节。如果结核性腱鞘炎和关节炎由于继发感染如金黄色葡萄球菌而变得复杂,可观察到严重的全身症状和关节损伤的增加。镰状细胞病和底部软骨细胞病以及其他关节受累和骨坏死的患者对结核病感染的易感性增加。此外,结核性关节炎的病例可见于干燥综合征、类风湿性关节炎、浆液性关节炎、痛风和Charcot关节病。免疫抑制和(或)糖皮质激素治疗,接受抗TNF治疗的患者已经提示关节感染的发生率增加。在低流行区和其他病理学病例中,由

于结核的诊断延迟，关节结核可导致关节严重变形和活动障碍。关节结核最常见于单关节。在不同的病例报告中，关于年龄和性别区别的研究结果有所不同。一般来说，结核性关节炎在儿童中更为常见。埃纳凯（Enache）等人在一份10年的病例报告中发现2/3的患者年龄超过40岁。在两项50年和60年的研究中报道了，女性的比率普遍更多；另外，在一些研究中发现，骨关节受累在男性中更为常见。

6.1.2 临床特点及诊断

肉芽肿样改变和软骨侵蚀导致了慢性积液和进行性关节损伤。急性炎症在骨关节结核中很少见，而局部畸形和活动受限更为常见。骨关节结核最常见的症状是慢性关节疼痛，它可能只是最轻微的炎症表现。在一些病例中，可以额外看到局部肿胀和窦道形成。单独关节的关节炎常见于骨关节结核。髋关节结核、膝关节结核和局部肌肉萎缩可能会引起一些畸形，并可能导致夜间强烈疼痛。发热、体重减轻和夜间盗汗等全身症状在结核性腱鞘炎和关节炎活动期间可能表现出来也可能不表现。不到50%的结核性腱鞘炎和关节炎患者患有活动性肺结核，但阴性结果不能排除诊断。虽然关节和肌腱的结核X线片影像学特征表现通常是非特异性的，但无痛性冷脓肿可能是唯一不常见的临床表现。影像学特征通常在发病的2～5个月后才能被识别出来。典型的结核性腱鞘炎和关节炎的影像学表现为关节旁骨质疏松、周围骨质疏松、关节内间隙逐渐狭窄。CT和MRI有助于进一步鉴别该病。MRI对软组织病变的诊断更好，而CT对骨损伤的诊断更好。结核性腱鞘炎和关节炎的MRI表现包括滑膜炎、渗出液、关节中央和周边侵蚀、活动性和慢性的血管痉挛、脓肿形成、骨折和低强度的滑膜炎。与X线片相比，MR也是非特异性的，但能更好地呈现病变范围。这些影像学特征可能有助于在适当的临床环境中诊断结核性腱鞘炎和关节炎。

严格的临床怀疑是必要的。在埃纳凯等人的病例研究中，临床上由于缺乏特异性临床表现而导致诊断关节结核感染的延误的病例有26%。另一方面，在一项回顾性评估中，只有26%的关节结核感染患者有提示性的临床表现。

临床上，结核病腱鞘炎和关节炎的评估分为5个阶段：

Ⅰ期或滑膜炎期：表现为组织水肿、骨损伤和局部骨质疏松，治疗效果良好；

Ⅱ期：表现为早期关节炎伴有边缘侵蚀（一个或多个侵蚀发生或骨质溶解性病变,关节间隙缩小）和轻度关节僵硬；

Ⅲ期：表现为晚期关节炎,伴有囊肿形成和关节间隙丧失；其结果是关节严重地丧失活动能力；

Ⅳ期：表现为关节炎处于较高水平,关节破坏有限,关节治疗后活动受限；

Ⅴ期：表现为关节强直。

一般的实验室检查表现既没有特异性也不可靠。可以观察到红细胞沉降率升高。结核菌素试验在高流行地区的成人中作用有限,但对5岁以下儿童有效。

滑膜液抽吸：滑膜液通常是非血性的,白细胞计数中等升高,不超过50 000个/ml,以多形白细胞或淋巴细胞为主。还应该计划做结核分枝杆菌的抗酸杆菌涂片和培养。滑膜液的直接涂片或手术标本抗酸杆菌检测最低在27%的病例中显示阳性。在抗酸杆菌检测中,建议至少有2个,最好是3个样本。如果样本中的细菌每毫升超过10 000个,则提示抗酸杆菌感染。

不同的培养方法,如Lowstein-Jensen培养基和放射性（Bactec 12B流体培养基）和无放射性（Bactec-MGIT-960系统）培养基可用于确认细菌缺乏状态。

诊断可分为三类：

1. 确诊结核——细菌培养阳性；
2. 疑似结核病——抗酸杆菌涂片阳性/慢性肉芽肿性炎症；
3. 可能是结核病——抗结核治疗后有良好的影像学表现和临床反应。

细菌细培养是金标准,标本为活检标本,关节腔抽吸或窦道标本应同时进行抗酸杆菌涂片和组织病理学检查。一般情况下,细菌培养阳性率较低。在这种情况下,组织病理学检查是重要的诊断检查之一。骨性病变/滑膜/软组织肿块的活检可能有助于避免诊断混乱。在资源有限的高流行地区,疑似诊断的患者可以通过临床特征和X线片报告来进行治疗,而无须活检。如果一个病例对化疗没有反应,并且怀疑有抗药性感染或其他疾病,建议进行滑膜活检。最重要的组织学评估结果是上皮样肉芽肿和干酪性坏死。在某些情况下,结核PCR阳性可能导致非特异性的肉芽肿反应。PCR技术可以提高敏感性,有助于排除软组织的非结核分枝杆菌感染。在一项研究中显示PCR的诊断率为33.3%。在由佐木(Sagoo)等人报告的肘关节结核病例中,当初始治疗不能完全缓解时,应进行滑膜活检并清创(连同涂片、细菌培养和PCR)。这可能是一个很好的诊断方法,但是昂贵和复杂,可能并不总是可行的。

早期诊断骨关节结核对防止晚期关节和骨结构破坏和全身播散感染具有重要意义。

结核菌素皮肤试验(tuberculin skin test,TST)是标准推荐的,但已知敏感性和特异性较低。如果结核病感染率很高,TST的阳性预测值将更高。此外,干扰素γ释放试验(IGRAs)是最近才出现的基于血液的检查,对慢性炎症性关节炎有很好的诊断价值,然而,其不确定的结果可能很难使用。

6.1.3　管理和治疗

夹板可以短暂地用于减轻急性症状,也可以在选定的病例中长时间使用,以防止感染的四肢和关节畸形。手术治疗通常是有限的,不必要的,除了活检以获得感染组织,开放或关节镜下清创,脓肿引流,滑膜切除术。然而,一些指征下,手术似乎是有益的。这些情况包括化疗没有反应,有持续感染,患者有反复发作的神经系统并发症。不建议对软骨严重破坏、畸形、大脓肿和耐多药结核的关节进行手术。

抗结核治疗是一种多种药物的复合治疗。治疗效果好,病死率低,即使在晚期的病例中,也可以看到良好的治疗反应。早期抗菌治疗可以近乎完全地治愈和功能关节保存。抗结核治疗一般持续至少9~12个月,但在儿童和免疫复合宿主中应持续更长时间。治疗肺结核的基本原则也适用于EPTB。除非已知或强烈怀疑对一线抗结核药物具有耐药性,通常初始治疗为服用异烟肼(isoniazid,INH)、利福平(rifampicin,RIF)、吡嗪酰胺(pyrazinamide,PZA)和乙胺丁醇(ethambutol,EMB)2个月,继续服用异烟肼和利福平7~10个月。

6.1.4　特殊关节感染

结核分枝杆菌引起的假关节感染(prosthetic joint infection,PJI)是罕见的,仅有很少的研究报道。一名误诊的患者在关节置换术后发生了膝或髋关节骨关节炎,并且培养阴性。对于组织学有肉芽肿病变特征,伴或不伴干酪性坏死,并且细菌培养阴性的假关节感染,诊断通常很困难,应该保持怀疑。可以通过在 Lowenstein 培养上分离微生物或通过分子技术(PCR)来证实诊断。人工关节置换术或人工关节融合术已被用于治疗 PJI,但当假体没有松动时,患者可以通过清创、在保留假体同时更换聚乙烯部分来治愈,并延长抗结核治疗(9～12个月)。

多灶性骨关节结核通常是 4～6 块骨头或关节受到影响,在一些病例里更集中。它主要发生在儿童手和脚上的扁骨,也可能有脊柱受累。全身显像可能有助于检测不同区域的病变。由于这种罕见的骨侵犯,临床上抗结核治疗的时间是不知道的,大多数患者治疗时间为 24 个月。

结核性骶髂炎有 4%～9.5% 的患者骶髂关节受累。诊断不能拖延(92%)。结核性骶髂关节炎可能与化脓性关节炎、炎症性疾病(如类风湿性关节炎)、强直性脊柱炎和 Reiter 病、肠道疾病和假移植物、肿瘤样疾病(如色素绒毛结节性滑膜炎)和地方性布鲁杆菌骶髂炎相混淆。关节融合术用于大的关节周围囊肿和持续疼痛的患者。这需要 6～9 个月的抗生素治疗。

6.2 结核性骨髓炎

6.2.1 流行病学

结核性骨髓炎约占所有 EPTB 病例的 10%,是胸膜和淋巴疾病后 EPTB 的第三种最常见类型。肺结核在很长一段时间内的表现可能是隐匿的,而且诊断可能是难以确定和存在延误的。这种诊断常与恶性肿瘤混淆。在一系列来自印度的 194 名结核病患者中,30% 的病例发生在 10～20 岁,22% 发生在 10 岁以内,18% 发生在 20～30 岁,14% 发生在 30～40 岁。结核性骨髓炎表现为双峰年龄分布:在发达国家,这种疾病通常影响 55 岁以上的人,而在移民中,这种疾病在年轻人中更常见(20～35 岁)。在骨骼结核患者中,有 6.9%～29% 的患者被诊断伴有肺部受累。

6.2.2 病理生理学

结核性骨髓炎的病理生理学通常是由首次感染时滞留在骨中的结核分

枝杆菌重新激活引起的。在成人中,病变可能是单一的,并影响任何骨骼,包括长骨、骨盆、肋骨和颅骨。在儿童中,主要为长骨的多处病变,但手脚的骨骼可能受累。

结核杆菌倾向脊柱和大关节,可以解释为脊椎和长骨生长板的血管供应丰富。结核性关节炎被认为是由骨骼中最早的传染性病灶延伸到关节所致。偶尔,结核杆菌可以沿着 Batson 椎旁静脉丛从肺到脊柱,或通过淋巴管引流到主动脉旁淋巴结。

骨关节病变是由原发性感染灶通过血行播散引起的。任何骨、关节或关节囊都可以被感染,但脊柱、骶髂关节和膝盖涵盖了 70%～80% 的感染,是感染好发部位。血行播散可发生在免疫功能低下的骨感染患者,如 HIV 患者或移植受者。

生长板(干骺端)接受最丰富的血液供应,通常是感染的初始部位。结核杆菌侵入末梢动脉,通过骨骺引起动脉炎和骨质破坏。细菌穿过骨骺后,可进入关节间隙,导致结核性关节炎,或从破坏的骨骼释放后形成窦道。M 型结核病不会产生任何破坏软骨的酶,就像化脓性感染一样。

可以出现一种闭合的囊性骨结核,尤其在长骨上,并且可能不像其他形式的骨结核那样有相关的硬化、骨质疏松或脓肿/窦道形成。这种形式的结核病更容易发生在儿童身上,并可能被误诊为恶性肿瘤。

如果得不到治疗感染进展,关节或骨周围的脓肿可能发展。这些通常被描述为"冷"脓肿,在愈合的病变中也经常出现钙化。随着感染面积的扩大,中心出现坏死,导致出现一个干酪样坏死区域。这种情况可能会导致骨扩张,并最终破坏骨皮质。没有骨再生(硬化)或骨膜反应是结核性骨髓炎常见的病理特征。

虽然不常见,结核病也可能涉及肋骨和头骨。颅骨几乎没有松质骨,通常受 M 型结核分枝杆菌的影响。累及颅骨的骨结核病通常发生在儿童身上,而且据说可能与头部外伤有关。

一些报告指出,创伤等机械因素与骨骼结核的发展之间存在关联。在加拿大对 99 例骨结核患者的一项研究中,30 例患者在患病前有外伤史,7 例患者近期有关节内类固醇注射的病史。这也可以解释为什么承重关节最易发生骨关节结核。创伤可能与骨结核有关,因为它导致血管增加,抵抗力下降,或暴露了潜伏的感染。

6.2.3　临床特征及诊断

结核性骨髓炎通常与结核性关节炎一起发生,但它可以作为一个独立疾病发生,没有关节受累。在成人中,没有关节受累的结核性骨髓炎通常表现为单个的病变,通常发生在长骨(如股骨和肱骨)的干骺端,尽管肋骨、骨盆、颅骨、乳突和下颌骨也可能受累。在儿童、老年人和免疫功能低下的人,包括感染 HIV 的人,病变可能是多个。在儿童中,病变可能影响手脚的短骨,有报告称结核性手足炎可以发生在成人中,但并不常见。病变广泛的患者可能被误诊为恶性肿瘤进展。细菌的重叠感染也可以掩盖诊断和表现,有报告称感染部位有金黄色葡萄球菌感染和结核病并存。结核性骨髓炎通常表现为骨旁疼痛和肿胀,最终限制患肢的活动。症状可能出现在诊断前的 6~24 个月。经常表现为发热、体重减轻和盗汗。通常在病程后期可能发生脓肿和窦道。颅骨结核性受累可能与头痛和软组织肿块有关。涉及肋骨的结核病表现为胸痛,有时伴有"冷"胸壁肿块。头颈部,特别是乳突和下颌骨的感染是由结核性中耳炎和口腔疾病引起的。面瘫可继发于结核性乳突炎。颞下颌关节结核也被报道为慢性颞下颌关节疼痛的原因。胸骨结核可表现为前胸痛。

诊断结核病需要很高的怀疑指数,特别是需要考虑到症状的潜在发作和从症状开始到疾病诊断之间的长期报告。在结核病发病率高的国家,根据临床和放射学检查,肌肉骨骼方面的主诉可能被正确地归因于结核病。在结核病发病率较低的发达国家,结核的诊断可能不会被首先考虑到,诊断经常被耽误。任何骨或关节都可能受累,但脊柱和负重关节是最常见的感染部位。疼痛是导致患者寻求医疗护理的最常见的主诉,在骨骼疼痛原因的鉴别诊断中应考虑结核病。有趣的是,局部疼痛、肿胀和活动受限有时甚至比放射线检查早 8 周。冷脓肿可能发生,有时伴有引流窦道,但这通常见于晚期、未经治疗的结核病或 HIV 感染患者中。结核性骨髓炎的鉴别诊断包括其他感染性原因导致的肌肉骨骼疾病(细菌、真菌和其他分枝杆菌致病原),以及恶性肿瘤、风湿性疾病和结节病。影像学技术,包括常规的 X 线片、CT 和 MRI,在评估疑似结核性骨髓炎和其他骨骼疾病的患者中是有用的。新技术的使用,如 CT、MRI 和 CT 引导下的细针穿刺活检技术彻底改变了诊断方法,与单纯的动脉造影和开放式活检相比,其结果更准确,侵入性更小。在此之前，常规影像学检查是结核性骨髓炎诊断的主要依据。

没有病理影像学表现，诊断通常是通过组织活检和(或)细菌培养。针吸和活检可以证实诊断与干酪性肉芽肿和抗酸杆菌(acid-fast bacilli, AFB)的存在。结核分枝杆菌培养阳性为结核性疾病提供了明确的证据，同时可以进行抗菌药物敏感性测试，这对于选择最佳治疗方案是必不可少的。对受累骨(通常是CT导向的)进行细针穿刺活检，以获得培养标本是有用的诊断方法。除了通过对受累组织活检获得的标本进行现代细菌培养技术外，使用分子诊断来检测结核分枝杆菌的存在有可能提高诊断骨结核和其他类型的肌肉和骨结核的能力。虽然对AFB涂片阳性的呼吸道标本进行核酸扩增，但关于这些检测数据对EPTB的作用有限。尤其是在结核性骨髓炎的分子诊断试验中。目前市面上可获得的和FDA批准的核酸扩增试验不被批准用于EPTB，包括结核性骨髓炎。虽然需要进一步的数据来证明这些测试在诊断结核性骨髓炎方面的效用，但是最近来自南非的报告感觉似乎很有希望，同时表明Xpert MTB/RIF可能是成人和儿童结核性骨髓炎的有价值的诊断试验。

最近由美国胸科学会、美国传染病学会和疾病预防控制中心发布的结核病诊断指南表明，对疑似EPTB患者的标本进行核酸扩增试验的数据质量较低；检测结果具有特异性，但可能缺乏敏感性。这表明，阳性Xpert MTB/RIF是有价值的，但阴性测试不排除EPTB。影像学上，结核性骨髓炎常与恶性肿瘤混淆，尤其是当病灶呈弥漫性和溶解性时。平片可显示骨质疏松、溶解、病变、硬化和骨膜炎。在破坏区域内，死骨可能表现为放射性增强的针状物。骨结核可见到囊性病变，尤其是儿童和年轻人。儿童的病变不如成人清楚，在成人中通常有明确的硬化边缘。多灶性疾病是一种罕见的表现，主要发生在儿童和免疫功能低下者。由于骨髓的改变，MRI在早期发现骨髓炎方面是有用的。结核性病变很少见于手和脚，但是结核性手足炎发生在儿童中是一个公认的结果。典型的放射学表现为"脊柱静脉"的气球状结构，骨溶解导致小梁吸收和受累手指扩张。

6.2.4 管理与治疗

没有对照试验评估结核性骨髓炎的治疗。根据治疗结核性脊椎炎的经验和治疗其他形式EPTB的经验，建议治疗药物敏感结核性骨髓炎可采用利福平为基础的短程治疗方案,就像用于治疗肺结核的那些方案。外科手术通常用于诊断,必要时可用于引流对药物治疗无效的脓肿或引流大脓肿以减轻张力。刮除和植骨,然后进行药物治疗,效果良好。晚期治疗或治疗不当会导致关节僵硬,纤维化或骨融合。目前还没有正式的指南,但一些专家建议,需要对静止性肺结核进行全关节置换的患者在术前至少3周和术后至少6~9个月接受围手术期化疗,以尽量减少复发的风险。对于药物敏感的骨结核的治疗,建议使用以利福平为基础的治疗方案,像治疗肺结核,共6~9个月。

6.3 结论

骨关节结核是一种非常罕见的结核病形式。据估计,骨关节结核约占所有结核病例的1.7%~2%。这种疾病的罕见性使普通医师对它的表现不太了解。因此,必须教育和提高所有医师对这种疾病表现的认识,以便及时诊断这种疾病。及时的诊断和治疗对于避免骨骼畸形的发展,最终避免长期功能障碍是非常重要的。新的成像方式的引入,包括MRI和CT,增强了对骨关节结核患者的诊断评估和对肌肉骨骼系统受累区域的直接活检。获得适当的标本进行培养和其他诊断检测是建立明确诊断和进行结核分枝杆菌药物敏感性测试的关键。

在所有患者中,64%~90%的患者可获得微生物和组织学阳性结果。研究表明,微生物检测不如关键性的活检敏感。总之,对影响身体任何部位的结核性骨髓炎和关节炎有较高的临床怀疑指数是很重要的。对怀疑有骨关节结核的患者应进行全面调查,必要时做活检。

参考文献

[1] Golden MP, Vikram HR. Extrapulmonary tuberculosis: an overview. Am Fam Physician. 2005; 72(9): 1761–1768.
[2] Malaviya AN, Kotwal PP. Arthritis associated with tuberculosis. Best Pract Res Clin Rheumatol. 2003; 17(2): 319–343.
[3] Tseng C, Huang RM, Chen KT. Tuberculosis arthritis: epidemiology, diagnosis, treatment. Clin Res Foot Ankle. 2014; 2: 131. https://doi.org/10.4172/2329-910X.1000131.
[4] Jutte PC, van Loenhout-Rooyackers JH, Borgdorff MW, van Horn JR. Increase

of bone and joint tuberculosis in the Netherlands. J Bone Joint Surg Br. 2004; 86: 901-904.
[5] Arathi N, Ahmad F, Huda N. Osteoarticular tuberculosis-a three years' retrospective study. J Clin Diagn Res. 2013; 10: 2189-2192.
[6] Haider ALM. Bones and joints tuberculosis. Bahrain Med Bull. 2007; 29: 1-9.
[7] Muangchan C, Nilganuwong S. The study of clinical manifestation of osteoarticular tuberculosis in Siriraj Hospital, Thailand. J Med Assoc Thail. 2009; 92: 101-109.
[8] Sagoo RS, Lakdawala A. Subbu tuberculosis of the elbow joint. J R Soc Med. 2011; 2: 17.
[9] Ruiz G, Rodriguez GJ, Guerri ML, Gonzalez A. Osteoarticular tuberculosis in a general hospital during the last decade. Clin Microbiol Infect. 2003; 9: 919-923.
[10] Enache SD, Pleasea IE, Anusca D, Zaharia B, Pop OT. Osteoarticular tuberculosis a ten years case review Rom. J Morphol Embryol. 2005; 46: 67-72.
[11] Grosskopf I, Ben David A, Charach G, Hochman I, Pitlik S. Bone and joint tuberculosis — a 10-year review. Isr J Med Sci. 1994; 30(4): 278-283.
[12] Pattamapaspong N, Muttarak M, Sivasomboon C. Tuberculosis arthritis and tenosynovitis. Semin Musculoskelet Radiol. 2011; 15(5): 459-469.
[13] Sharma SK, Mohan A. Extrapulmonary tuberculosis. Indian J Med Res. 2004; 120: 316-353.
[14] Triplett D, Stewart E, Mathew S, Horne BR, Prakash V. Delayed diagnosis of tuberculous arthritis of the knee in an air force service member: case report and review of the literature. Mil Med. 2016; 181(3): e306-309.
[15] Chen SC, Chen KT. Updated diagnosis and management of osteoarticular tuberculosis. J Emerg Med Trauma Surg Care. 2014; 1: 002.
[16] Narang S. Tuberculosis of the entheses. Int Orthop. 2012; 36: 2373-2378.
[17] Gehlot PS, Chaturvedi S, Kashyap R, Singh V. Pott's spine: retrospective analysis of MRI scans of 70 cases. J Clin Diagn Res. 2012; 6: 1534-1538.
[18] Sawlani V, Chandra T, Mishra RN, Aggarwal A, Jain UK, Gujral RB. MRI features of tuberculosis of peripheral joints. Clin Radiol. 2003; 58(10): 755-762.
[19] Spiegel DA, Singh GK, Banskota AK. Tuberculosis of the musculoskeletal system. Tech Orthop. 2005; 20: 167-178.
[20] Titov AG, Vyshnevskaya EB, Mazurenko SI, Santavirta S, Konttinen YT. Use of polymerase chain reaction to diagnose tuberculous arthritis from joint tissues and synovial fluid. Arch Pathol Lab Med. 2004; 28: 205-209.
[21] Araujo Z, de Waard JH, de Larrea CF, Borges R, Convit J. The effect of Bacille Calmette-Guérin vaccine on tuberculin reactivity in indigenous children from communities with high prevalence of tuberculosis. Vaccine. 2008; 26: 5575-5581.
[22] Song SE, Yang J, Lee KS, Kim H, Kim YM, Kim S, Park MS, Oh SY, Lee JB, Lee E, Park SH, Kim HJ. Comparison of the tuberculin skin test and interferon gamma release assay for the screening of tuberculosis in adolescents in close contact with tuberculosis TB patients. PLoS One. 2014; 9(7): e100267.
[23] Chen SH, Lee CH, Wong T, Feng HS. Long-term retrospective analysis of surgical treatment for irretrievable tuberculosis of the ankle. Foot Ankle Int.

2013; 34(3): 372-379.
[24] Lawn SD, Zumla AI. Tuberculosis. Lancet. 2011; 378(9785): 57-72.
[25] Pigrau-Serrallach C, Rodríguez-Pardo D. Bone and joint tuberculosis. Eur Spine J. 2013; 22(4): 556-566.
[26] Shanbhag V, Kotwal R, Gaitonde A, Singhal K. Total hip replacement infected with Mycobacterium tuberculosis. A case report with review of literature. Acta Orthop Belg. 2007; 73(2): 268-274.
[27] Leonard MK, Blumberg HM. Musculoskeletal tuberculosis. Microbiol Spectr. 2017; 5(2).
[28] Gunal S, Yang Z, Agarwal M, Koroglu M, Arici ZK, Durmaz R. Demographic and microbial characteristics of extrapulmonary tuberculosis cases diagnosed in Malatya, Turkey, 2001-2007. BMC Public Health. 2011; 11: 154-161.
[29] Gardam M, Lim S. Mycobacterial osteomyelitis and arthritis. Infect Dis Clin N Am. 2005; 19: 819-830.
[30] Held MFG, Hoppe S, Laubscher M, Mears S, Dix-Peek S, Zar HJ, Dunn RN. Epidemiology of musculoskeletal uberculosis in an area with high disease prevalence. Asian Spine J. 2017; 11(3): 405-411.
[31] Rosli FJ, Haron R. Tuberculosis of the skull mimicking a bony tumor. Asian J Neurosurg. 2016; 11(1): 68.
[32] Prakash J, Vijay V. Tuberculosis of the patella imitating chronic knee synovitis. BMJ Case Rep. 2014; 15: 2014.
[33] Jurado LF, Murcia MI, Hidalgo P, Leguizamón JE, González LR. Phenotypic and genotypic diagnosis of bone and miliary tuberculosis in an HIV+ patient in Bogotá, Colombia. Biomedica. 2015; 35(1): 8-15.
[34] Chen ST, Zhao LP, Dong WJ, Gu YT, Li YX, Dong LL, Ma YF, Qin SB, Huang HR. The clinical features and bacteriological characterizations of bone and joint tuberculosis in China. Sci Rep. 2015; 8(5): 11084.
[35] Epperla N, Kattamanchi S, Fritsche TR. Appearances are deceptive: Staphylococcus superinfection of clavicular tuberculous osteomyelitis. Clin Med Res. 2015; 13(2): 85-88.
[36] Izawa K, Kitada S. Clinical analysis of osteoarticular nontuberculous mycobacterial infection. Kekkaku. 2016; 91(1): 1-8.
[37] Hand JM, Pankey GA. Tuberculous otomastoiditis. Microbiol Spectr. 2016; 4(6): 1-2.
[38] Assouan C, Anzouan K, Nguessan ND, Millogo M, Horo K, Konan E, Zwetyenga N. Tuberculosis of the temporomandibular joint. Rev Stomatol Chir Maxillofac Chir Orale. 2014; 115(2): 88-93.
[39] Cataño JC, Galeano D, Botero JC. Tuberculous sternal osteomyelitis. Am J Emerg Med. 2014; 32(10): 1302.
[40] Prakash M, Gupta P, Sen RK, Sharma A, Khandelwal N. Magnetic resonance imaging evaluation of tubercular arthritis of the ankle and foot. Acta Radiol. 2015; 56(10): 1236-1241.
[41] Colmenero JD, Ruiz-Mesa JD, Sanjuan-Jimenez R, Sobrino B, Morata P. Establishing the diagnosis of tuberculous vertebral osteomyelitis. Eur Spine J.

2013; 22(Suppl 4): 579-586.
[42] Watt JP, Davis JH. Percutaneous core needle biopsies: the yield in spinal tuberculosis. S Afr Med J. 2013; 104(1): 29-32.
[43] Gu Y, Wang G, Dong W, Li Y, Ma Y, Shang Y, Qin S, Huang H. Xpert MTB/RIF and genotype MTBDR plus assays for the rapid diagnosis of bone and joint tuberculosis. Int J Infect Dis. 2015; 36: 27-30.
[44] Held M, Laubscher M, Mears S, Dix-Peek S, Workman L, Zar H, Dunn R. Diagnostic accuracy of the Xpert MTB/RIF assay for extrapulmonary tuberculosis in children with musculoskeletal infections. Pediatr Infect Dis J. 2016; 35: 1165-1168.
[45] Lewinsohn DM, Leonard MK, LoBue PA, Cohn DL, Daley CL, Desmond E, Keane J, Lewinsohn DA, Loeffler AM, Mazurek GH, O'Brien RJ, Pai M, Richeldi L, Salfinger M, Shinnick TM, Sterling TR, Warshauer DM, Woods GL. Official American Thoracic Society/Infectious Diseases Society of America/Centers for Disease Control and Prevention clinical practice guidelines: diagnosis of tuberculosis in adults and children. Clin Infect Dis. 2017; 64: 111-115.
[46] Hu S, Guo J, Ji T, Shen G, Kuang A. Multifocal osteoarticular tuberculosis of the extremities in an immunocompetent young man without pulmonary disease: a case report. Exp Ther Med. 2015; 9(6): 2299-2302.
[47] Morris BS, Varma R, Garg A, Awasthi M, Maheshwari M. Multifocal musculoskeletal tuberculosis in children: appearances on computed tomography. Skelet Radiol. 2002; 31: 1-8.
[48] Sarkar AS, Garg AK, Bandyopadhyay A, Kumar S, Pal S. Tuberculosis of distal radius presenting as cystic lesion in a nine-month-old infant: a rare case report. J Clin Diagn Res. 2016; 10(9): 6-7.
[49] Kadu VV, Saindane KA, Godghate N, Godghate NN. Tuberculosis of calcaneum a rare presentation. J Orthop Case Rep. 2016; 6: 61-62.
[50] Mariconda M, Cozzolino A, Attingenti P, Cozzolino F, Milano C. Osteoarticular tuberculosis in a developed country. J Infect. 2007; 54: 375-380.

7
结核性脊椎炎

艾塞·巴蒂雷尔

7.1 导论与流行病学

根据 WHO 的《2016 年全球结核病报告》,全球估计新增结核病病例为 1 040 万(其中 56% 为男性),2015 年估计因结核病死亡的人数为 140 万。同年,结核病仍然位居全球十大死因之列。"结核性脊椎椎间盘炎""脊柱结核"和"Pott 病"是指结核分枝杆菌感染脊椎的同义词,非结核分枝杆菌(NTM)很少引起脊椎骨髓炎[1,2]。在罗伯特·科赫(Robert Koch)于 1882 年描述结核杆菌之前,Pott 病(Pott's disease)于 1779 年由佩西瓦尔·波特爵士(Sir Perciall Pott)根据一名脊柱畸形和截瘫患者的临床表现首次定义[3]。肌肉和骨结核约占 EPTB 病例的 10%,占所有结核病病例的 1%~5%[1,4-6]。脊柱结核是最常见的骨结核(约占总病例数的 50%),其次是结核性关节炎和椎外结核性骨髓炎[7-10]。男性人群患脊柱结核的风险稍高一些,半数以上的患者是男性[11]。患者年龄 8~60 岁,平均 40~50 岁。在流行地区,多发生于较年幼的患儿中,而在非流行地区,它主要发生在成人中[11,12]。脊柱结核是大多数发展中国家的地方病。在 10 年间(从 2002 年到 2011 年),脊柱结核在美国的发病率显著下降。尽管并不常见,脊柱结核仍然是一个公共卫生问题[13]。近几十年来,由于 HIV 感染患者、来自结核病流行国家的移民[11],与结核病总发病率相比,发达国家的结核病发病率一直在上升。HIV 感染患者的脊柱结核发生率与未感染 HIV 的患者相当[1,12,14]。脊柱结核的历史可以追溯到骨骼受损的埃及木乃伊,结核分枝杆菌复合体 DNA 在木乃伊的骨损标本中被检测到证实了这一点[15-17]。

脊柱结核是一个严重的公共卫生问题,因为这种破坏性形式的结核病的诊断通常会因为其缓慢的病程而延误。延误诊断和治疗会导致永久性后遗症,如畸形和神经功能障碍[1]。尽管在诊断工具和治疗方面取得了进步,但脊柱结核仍然是 21 世纪发病率和病死率较高的疾病之一[18]。

7.2 病因学和病理生理学

在原发感染过程中,结核杆菌通过血源性播散到骨骼。局部获得性免疫反应在一定程度上限制了原发感染灶。通过淋巴引流从原发病灶向周围扩散或通过淋巴引流发展为感染是非常罕见的。结核的易感条件,如免疫抑制、高龄、HIV 感染、营养不良或慢性肾衰竭,可能导致椎骨中这些病灶的潜伏感染重新激活[19,20]。骨髓炎和关节炎都发生在脊柱结核。结核杆菌最初的感染部位是骺板,之后是椎间关节炎症,然后感染扩散到相邻的两个椎体[21],侵入末梢动脉会导致骨质破坏,在椎间盘连续受累的情况下,就像所谓的脊椎椎间盘炎一样,可能会发生椎体塌陷。有时,无血管椎间盘可以幸免于难,在这种情况下,"脊柱炎"的诊断是首选的。脊椎结构周围可能会形成冷性脓肿。感染灶引流到腰肌会引起肌炎,然后可能发展成腰大肌脓肿。干扰素-γ、$CD4^+$ 和 $CD8^+$ T 淋巴细胞是结核细胞免疫反应的重要因素[22]。在感染灶的组织病理标本中,除淋巴细胞外,还可见上皮样组织细胞、巨细胞、浆细胞和成纤维细胞。局部病理反应可见有渗出性干酪样坏死破坏骨组织以及肉芽组织增生。愈合过程通常伴随着纤维组织的形成和钙化。与化脓性骨髓炎不同,脊柱结核不发生骨膜反应或硬化性骨再生[23]。大多数情况下,椎体的前部受累[24]。椎体前部塌陷导致"gibbus 畸形"(与 Pott 病相关的后凸畸形)。脊柱结核最常累及胸椎和腰椎[25,26]。

7.3 临床表现

临床表现隐匿,疾病早期无明显症状[1]。在一项包括 314 名脊柱结核患者的多国多中心研究发现,从症状出现到诊断的中位持续时间接近 2.5 个月[27]。在另一项来自欧洲的研究中,诊断前症状持续时间的中位数为 4 个月[28]。最常见的症状是背部疼痛或受累部位疼痛[12]。疼痛的严重程度随着时间的推移而增加。受累椎骨周围可能会发生肌肉痉挛。发热、体重减轻和盗汗等症状较少见,只有不到一半的患者出现,在晚期疾病中更为常见[29]。但是,在中国报告的入组人数最多的 967 例脊柱结核患者中,继发于腰痛后常见的症状是发热和盗汗[26]。体格检查时,可出现棘突局部压痛,活动范围试验引起的剧烈疼痛,晚期可出现脊柱后凸和神经症状,如麻木、刺痛、虚弱,甚至截瘫。在最大的病例系列中,来自中国的 967 名脊柱结核患者中,有 1/3 的患者有神经受累[26]。在法国进行的另一项研究中,50%的患者有神经系统症状和体征[28]。王华等人研究了 329 名脊柱结核患者发现,患者发生感觉和运动障碍的概率分别为 54%和 28%[30]。如果能在出现时早期诊断并及时进行紧急减压治疗,神经功能障碍通常是可逆的[31]。这种疾病的典型表现包括背部疼痛、吉布斯畸形或截瘫。不典型的表现包括硬膜外脓肿,无明显前椎受累,脊柱多节段不毗连,双侧腰肌脓肿,仅累及脊柱后段,以及骶部脊柱结核[32-34]。

胸椎是最常见的受累部位,其次是腰椎和颈椎,发生病变概率呈递减趋势[12]。在巴基斯坦的一个大型病例研究报道,受累椎体节段的频率为胸椎(45%),其次是腰骶椎(33%)、颈椎(10%)和多节段(12%)[11]。夏尔马·A(Sharma A)等对 312 例脊柱结核患者的临床特点进行了分析,他们发现胸椎最常受累(46%),其次是胸腰椎椎骨(28%)。在 80%的患者中,只有 1~2 个相邻的椎骨受累[35],而在免疫功能低下的患者(如 HIV 感染者)中,可能会看到多发性脊椎病变。非结核分枝杆菌感染通常在老年和(或)免疫抑制患者中表现为脊柱广泛分布的病变[36]。作为脊柱结核的病因,分离到的最常见的非结核分枝杆菌是禽类分枝杆菌复合体(M. avium complex, MAC),其次是异种分枝杆菌,与 HIV 感染无关。在 HIV 感染的患者中,非结核分枝杆菌引起的脊柱结核发生的年龄较小,一半的非结核分枝杆菌引起的脊柱结核患者存在多种形式的免疫抑制,而 15%的患者有手术史或外伤史,这些患者中有 2/3 需要手术治疗[37]。

神经症状发生于颈椎脊柱结核的病程早期[38]。咽后壁脓肿可能是颈椎脊柱结核的临床表现[2,39]。QuantiFERON(®)- TB Gold 试管试验是一种干扰素-γ 释放试验(interon-gamma releases assay, IGRA),在 75%的患者中呈阳性[40],合并肺结核病例有 3%~14%[26,27,31]。因此,胸片对脊柱结核的诊断并不十分有意义,但为了排除肺结核,应该始终进行检测,因为肺结核需要隔离痰涂片抗酸杆菌(acido-resistant bacilli, ARB)阳性的患者。此外,肺部受累可能有助于脊柱结核的诊断。

7 结核性脊椎炎

由于延误诊断,椎体塌陷可能导致脊柱后凸或"gibbus 畸形",这是结构性后凸的一种形式,可能会导致脊髓受压。截瘫的原因是脊髓受压,可能是由于因为 gibbus 畸形所导致,也可能是因为骨赘。40%～70%的病例在诊断时可能已经存在脊髓压迫[41]。脊柱结核最常见的并发症是截瘫和四肢瘫痪,这取决于受累脊柱水平的神经根和脊柱畸形(脊柱后凸或脊柱侧凸)。未经治疗的病例也可能发生压缩性骨折。引起脊柱半脱位的臂骨畸形可能会由于脊髓受压而导致神经功能障碍。如果在表现时有任何运动障碍,即使接受治疗也不太可能完全恢复。

椎旁"冷脓肿"(软组织肿块)比较常见于脊柱结核,椎旁脓肿可能发生钙化。腰大肌可能因结核杆菌感染的扩散而受累[7]。在结核病流行国家,结核分枝杆菌是腰肌脓肿的一种相当常见的病因。与布鲁辛斯基征和化脓性脊椎骨髓炎相比,脊柱结核更常导致神经功能障碍、脊柱畸形和椎旁脓肿。此外,在脊柱结核[42]中,胸椎更常受累。未累及椎间盘的非连续多节段椎体受累是脊柱结核的一种非典型形式,相当罕见(3%～16%)[11,26,27,43,44],其临床表现类似于恶性疾病[32,44]。

表 7-1 列出了脊柱结核的症状和体征及其发生概率。

表 7-1 脊柱结核的症状和体征[1,3,27,28]

	发生概率(%)
慢性背痛	58～87
局部脊柱压痛	21
发热	31～48
体重减轻	41～48
盗汗	18～49
冷脓肿	69
脊柱旁	59～63
腰大肌	22～29
脊柱后凸/吉布斯畸形	46
神经功能障碍	40～56
下肢无力	69
截瘫	10～25
脊柱失稳	21～33

7.4 诊断

由于临床表现不典型,脊柱结核诊断通常会被延误。需要及时诊断,及时开始适当的治疗,以防止永久性后遗症的发生发展。因此,基于流行病学、既往病史和(或)接触史、临床线索和特征性影像学表现的脊柱结核的高度怀疑指数在早期诊断中至关重要[1,12]。特别是在 HIV 感染的患者中,可能没有其他症状或体征。在结核病流行的国家,骨骼疼痛可能会导致在最初表现时考虑脊柱结核。然而,在结核病发病率较低的发达国家,诊断可能会被忽视和延误。

影像学手段(X 线片、CT 和 MRI)是判断脊柱结核的有用方式。在病程早期,X 线片对诊断不敏感。影像病理发现,脊柱结核首先发生在反应性硬化症椎体的前部,椎体终板变得脱矿[45],随后邻近椎骨受累导致前楔形。脓肿中的钙化也可以在 X 线片上显示[46],但是,在脊柱结核病程的早期,X 线片检查对诊断没有太大的意义[47]。CT 可显示骨硬化和破坏、椎间盘溶解和塌陷、邻近椎体破坏、硬膜外延伸(超过 60% 的患者存在)和脓肿钙化[48,49]。CT 对细针穿刺引流和经皮穿刺引流也有一定的指导意义。CT 引导下骨活检对脊柱结核的诊断阳性率为 60%~80%,与手术活检相当[28,50]。CT 引导下活检对硬膜外浸润和椎旁脓肿的特异性分别为 83% 和 91%[51]。

MRI 是诊断脊柱结核最敏感的影像学检查方法。MRI 上所见的椎体前部破坏、椎体前楔形和椎旁冷性脓肿有利于脊柱结核的诊断[11,46]。增强 MRI 还能显示神经根或脊髓受压[52,53]。MRI 在脊柱结核的诊断中优于其他影像学检查,因为它具有高对比度软组织分辨率、多平面成像和高灵敏度来发现早期骨髓浸润[11]。在 T1 加权像上,可以显示脊椎骨髓低信号、椎间盘高度降低、椎旁软组织肿块和炎症的硬膜外侵犯。在 T2 加权图像上,受累的椎体、椎间盘和软组织显示为等信号或高信号区域[11]。大多数(85%)的患者有典型的 MRI 表现[35]。MRI 上的硬膜外/椎旁脓肿通常更倾向于结核性脊柱炎而不是化脓性脊柱炎[54,55]。脊柱结核的影像学特征总结见表 7-2。三个不同的 Pott 病患者的 MRI 图像如图(图 7-1、图 7-2 和图 7-3)所示。

7 结核性脊椎炎

表 7-2 结核性脊柱炎的影像学表现[42,46]

影像学表现
邻近椎体受累
累及多个椎体节段
椎体终板脱矿
椎体前部溶解性破坏
残留椎间盘
由于椎间盘损坏而导致的椎间盘狭窄
椎体前楔形
椎体塌陷
感染的韧带下播散
椎旁脓肿
腰大肌受累或脓肿
MRI不均匀信号强度与边缘强化

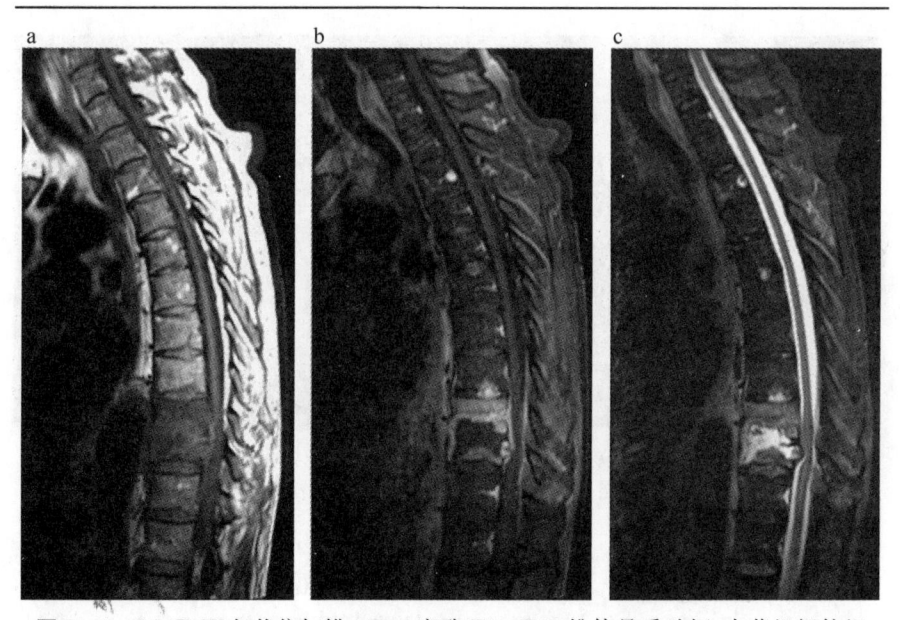

图 7-1 (a) T1W矢状位扫描：Pott病致T10、T11椎体骨质破坏，肉芽组织软组织向椎旁延伸，T10~T11椎体间有骨内脓肿，破坏终板。破坏的T11椎体后缘膨出，椎管狭窄，脊髓受压明显。(b) T1W矢状位图像（增强后）：T10和T11椎体可见Pott病破坏性病变增强。(c) T2W矢状位扫描：典型T10、T11椎体骨质破坏，软组织成分向椎旁延伸，T10~T11椎体间可见脓肿，破坏终板。由于破坏的T11椎体后缘膨出，也有椎管狭窄和脊髓受压（压缩性脊髓病）

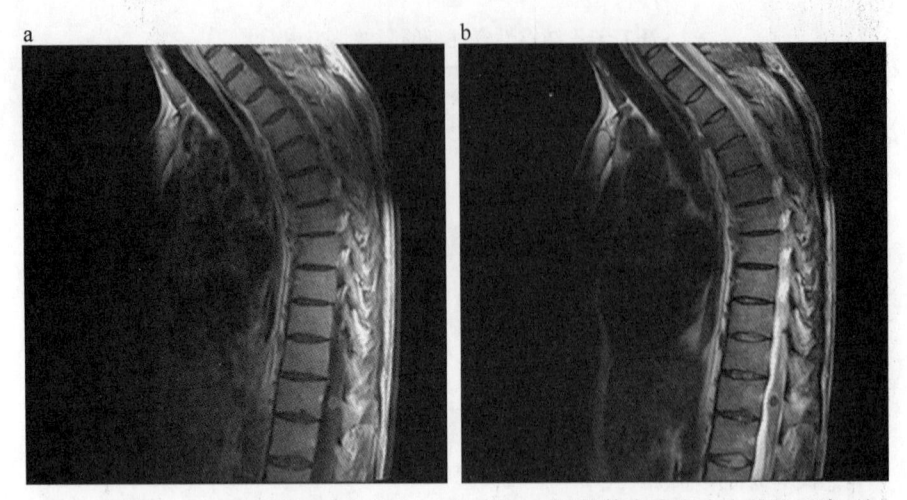

图7-2 （a）T1W矢状图（对比度后）。由于Pott病，椎体高度有多个节段下降，关节间隙变窄。T11椎体水平的脊髓远端可见脊柱结核瘤。增强后序列图像表现为周边对比度增强。（b）T2W矢状位扫描：T11椎体水平的脊柱结核瘤，中心呈低信号，外围呈高信号

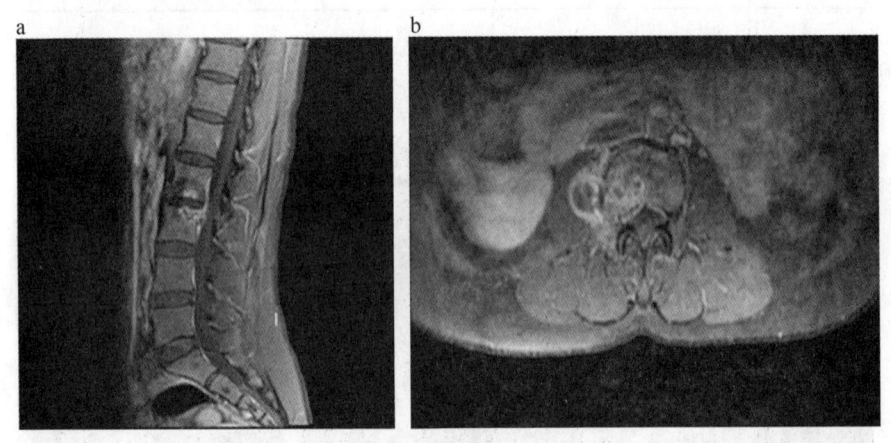

图7-3 （a）T1W矢状位扫描：Pott病累及L2、L3椎体和L2、L3椎间盘终板和椎体。（b）T1W轴位增强扫描：右椎旁可见继发于腰椎Pott病的腰大肌脓肿，周围有增强

脊柱结核可以通过CT或超声引导的细针穿刺活检（fine-needle aspiration and biopsy，FNAB）获得的受累组织和骨骼受累部分的微生物学和（或）组织病理学检查来确诊[52]。然而，在27%的病例中FNAB不足以诊断[56]。微生物学检查包括抗酸杆菌（acid-fast bacillus，AFB）染色标本显微镜检查和分枝杆菌培养。如果能获得合适的标本，可以在1/3的患者中明确微生物学诊断[12]。如果能在结核培养中分离出分枝杆菌，药敏试验对于得出最

佳治疗方案至关重要[57-59]。从鼻窦窦道中培养出的菌落可能显示有定殖微生物。获得深部骨或软组织是正确诊断病因所必需的。如果CT或超声引导的FNAB显示干酪性肉芽肿和AFB，则脊柱结核可以确诊。其他肉芽肿性疾病如布鲁氏菌病、真菌感染、非结核分枝杆菌感染等在脊柱结核的鉴别诊断中应予以考虑。虽然目前FDA没有批准用于EPTB，但分子诊断方法（如核酸扩增）可以用来提高诊断概率。分子诊断法提高了肌肉骨骼结核的诊断率，尽管有较高的诊断特异性[59-61]，但缺乏敏感性。此外，在结核病高度流行的国家，用于检测核酸和利福平耐药性的快速自动化生长系统和分子测试（如Xpert MTB/RIF分析）的可用性仍然有限[60]。Xpert MTB/RIF试验的敏感性和特异性分别为62%和100%[62]。在结核病高度流行且资源有限的国家，脊柱结核的诊断通常基于流行病学、临床和影像学特征。与其他形式的骨髓炎一样，80%以上的患者红细胞沉降率（erythrocyte sedimentation rate，ESR）普遍升高[63]。

7.5 鉴别诊断

脊柱结核的鉴别诊断包括由布鲁菌属、念珠菌属、其他地方性真菌、放线菌属、类鼻疽伯克霍尔德菌属和一些细菌如金黄色葡萄球菌引起的其他亚急性或慢性脊椎肉芽肿和非肉芽肿感染[64]。在传染病病原学的鉴别诊断中应考虑流行病学特征。与布鲁型脊柱炎相比，脊柱结核表现为需要手术引流的化脓性脓肿形成以及更常见的脊柱并发症[65]。

非感染性疾病，如脊椎关节病、退行性变、椎体骨质疏松性塌陷、创伤性骨折，特别是原发性或转移性恶性肿瘤，可能与脊柱结核的表现相似[7,66]。

7.6 治疗

脊柱结核治疗的主要目标是立即缓解症状（疼痛、下肢轻瘫和截瘫），恢复神经和运动功能，防止永久性后遗症，以及根除感染。早期诊断、及时治疗，并给予适当的抗结核药物治疗，可防止神经功能障碍、脊柱畸形等后遗症的发生。针对药物敏感或耐药分枝杆菌的肺结核病治疗原则也适用于EPTB[67]。英国医学研究理事会小组已经定义了脊柱结核的现代管理策略，该小组进行了脊柱结核患者的随机试验[68]。大量患者参加了这些试验，但由于颈椎脊柱结核的发病率较低，因此没有纳入为研究对象，对颈部脊柱结核患者的治疗建议大多基于病例系列研究[69-71]。以利福平为基础的较长疗程的抗结核治疗加上有适应证的前路手术，使得大多数颈椎脊柱结核患者完全康复。椎板切除术在缓解颈髓压迫方面效果不佳。此外，由于颈椎失稳的风险，不推荐使用椎板切除术[69]。此外，脊髓病患者也被排除在外。然而，在另一项研究中，对于功能性或完全缓解脊髓病来说，药物治疗即可[72]。

抗结核药物治疗

对于大多数没有任何神经功能障碍的患者来说，仅用抗结核药物就足够了。标准的抗结核药物组合异烟肼、利福平和吡嗪酰胺，加或不加乙胺丁醇6个月、9个月或12个月，并在有适应证的情况下进行手术，构成了脊柱结核的主要治疗方法。抗结核（抗结核）药物方案的选择因分枝杆菌是否具有抗药性以及患者是否感染 HIV 而有所不同。抗结核治疗的最佳持续时间是不确定的，取决于分离的分枝杆菌的敏感性和抗结核药物方案的组成。

长程疗法（12～18个月）已被推荐用于脊柱结核。然而，研究表明，以利福平为基础的一线抗结核药物（即异烟肼＋利福平6个月，链霉素前3个月）联合手术切除和植骨治疗6～9个月，对易感分枝杆菌且治疗反应良好的患者已足够[7,73,74]。根治性清创手术后6个月、9个月和18个月的方案都有类似的结果。在接受三种方案中的任何一种的患者中都没有观察到结核病的复发或再燃[73]。在选定的接受手术干预（包括彻底清创、植骨和内固定）的患者中，即使是4.5个月的超短程治疗也和9个月的治疗一样获得了较好的疗效[75]。

相比之下，一项回顾性研究报告了抗结核治疗6个月的复发率很高（62%），而抗结核治疗9个月的疗程没有观察到复发[74]。对于治疗反应差、耐多药结核病（MDR-TB）的晚期病例，需要进行9～12个月的治疗[67,76]。骨关节多药耐药结核（MDR-TB）在医学文献中很少有报道。如果这些病例有适应证，二线抗结核药物和手术可以获得良好的临床效果[77]。

对于胸腰椎交界处脊柱结核椎体高度毁损50%以上及疼痛剧烈的患者，建议采用卧床和（或）石膏/矫形器固定。康斯塔姆（Konstam）和布莱索夫斯基（Blesovsky）报告了一种不需要固定或支撑的门诊治疗方法，即通过至少12个月疗程的异烟肼和对氨基水杨酸（p-aminosalicylic acid，PAS）的药物治疗脊柱结核[78]，只有一小部分需要脓肿引流的患者进行了手术，86%的患者仅通过药物治疗就可以完全康复。

美国疾病控制与预防中心(CDC)、美国传染病学会(IDSA)和美国胸科学会(ATS)的脊柱结核治疗指南建议在简单病例中使用药物而不是手术治疗[67]，因为在简单病例中，外科清创结合药物治疗并不比单独使用药物治疗更具有优势[72,79]。在一项系统回顾和荟萃分析中，近30%的药物治疗脊髓硬膜外脓肿失败的患者需要手术治疗[80]。

手术治疗

需要手术的患者百分比存在个体性差异[12]。约有2/3~3/4的患者可能需要手术[26,81]。其中1/3的患者仅实施内科治疗，其余2/3的患者需要诊断性和(或)治疗性手术干预[27]。

手术适应证包括初诊时脊柱后凸＞40°(使用改良的Konstam法从脊柱侧位X线片测量脊柱后凸角度)或进行性后凸，晚期病例因脊髓受压而导致的神经功能障碍，尽管适当治疗仍有神经功能障碍的进展(持续恶化)、对化疗反应差、冷脓肿引流、脊柱失稳，以及诊断目的并非为获得细针穿刺结果的患者。急性神经损伤和脊柱失稳的患者应及早手术。在临床和神经功能正常的患者中，手术治疗可能会延后[67,68,82-85]。

外科治疗脊柱结核的目的是清除感染组织，减轻疼痛，通过减压和脊柱稳定来改善神经功能障碍，纠正畸形和恢复功能[1]。手术治疗包括清除感染物质、引流脓肿(如果有)、减压、植骨和使用硬件固定脊柱[85,86]。根据椎体的不同部位和椎体水平，无论是否存在冷脓肿，已经描述了不同的手术入路[87-89]。在疾病的早期阶段，后路用五金器械固定，以防止后凸畸形。一些在病程后期出现脊柱畸形的病例首选前路手术，以防止畸形的进展[68]。霍奇森(Hodgson)等人报道了采用前路手术切除减压、自体骨移植和抗结核治疗的成功率[90]。在某些情况下，在完成抗结核治疗后，可能需要进行脊柱畸形(例如，脊柱后凸)的重建手术。可能需要使用硬件来稳定脊柱[89]。有神经症状和(或)胸椎或腰椎破坏性骨损伤的患者可能受益于微创外科干预措施，如电视胸腔镜前路手术[91,92]。在治疗累及骨骼其他部位的肌肉骨骼结核时，手术的必要性值得商榷[79]。因此，并不是所有的脊柱结核病例都需要常规手术[93,94]。

神经运动障碍分为四级：1级，可忽略；2级，轻度；3级，中度；4级，严重(包括感觉和自主神经功能障碍)。1级和2级推荐保守治疗；4级推荐手术治疗。3级患者仍处于灰色地带,对治疗方式的决定尚未达成共识[95]。

HIV 阴性和 HIV 感染患者的脊柱结核管理策略没有区别[95],但是,对于同时接受脊柱结核的抗结核治疗和 HIV 感染的抗逆转录病毒治疗(antiretroviral treatment,ART)的 HIV 感染患者,强烈建议对免疫重建炎症综合征(immure reconstitution inflammatory syndrome,IRIS)进行监测。在开始抗逆转录病毒治疗后,结核病临床和实验室结果的矛盾进展应警惕 IRIS 的发生,IRIS 患者会表现出新的临床表现和(或)影像学表现,或再现已缓解的体征或症状[96,97]。

对于胸腰椎脊柱结核的外科治疗,前入路或后入路可能是首选的,但后外侧入路可以更好地矫正后凸角度和改善背部疼痛[98]。然而,后外侧手术花费更多的手术时间,导致更多的出血和术后窦道形成[99-101]。此外,后路手术没有改善的患者可能需要前路手术[88]。对于胸腰椎脊柱结核的治疗,一期经椎弓根清创、后路内固定和融合术已被报道为有效的,术后长期效果令人满意[102]。在单节段脊柱结核患者中,使用钛网笼的临床效果与自体髂骨移植相当。它们还可用于多节段脊柱结核的外科治疗,具有良好的临床疗效[103]。在有多节段相邻椎体受累的胸椎脊柱结核,后路内固定更有利于持久矫正脊柱后凸[99]。同样,后路手术入路是治疗腰骶段脊柱结核的有效方法[104,105]。

对治疗反应的监测通过症状和体征的缓解以及感觉和运动神经功能的改善来评估临床反应。炎症标志物如 C 反应蛋白、红细胞沉降率在评价治疗反应方面的作用有限。术后 6 周内连续红细胞沉降率测定减少 2/3 和 C 反应蛋白水平降低可能表明对治疗的良好反应和迅速的神经恢复[106]。尽管进行了适当的治疗,但放射学结果可能在病程中延迟表现出来,甚至可能观察到进展。因此,不建议进行重复的系列成像研究[107]。轻度虚弱,肌力改善,较低的截瘫评分,感觉诱发电位(SEPs)和运动诱发电位(MEPs)是波特病截瘫患者 6 个月良好预后的预测因子[108]。对患者的随访应持续到治疗结束后至少 1～5 年,以确定治疗的长期结果。

7.7 预后

脊柱结核的乐观结局可以定义为"随着疾病的临床症状和影像学结果的改善,骨骼活动充分自如,没有功能障碍"。脊椎受累程度、患者入院时的美国脊髓损伤协会损伤分级(AIS 分级)以及膀胱和肠道受累显著影响神经功能改善的最终结果[35]。

图尔古特·M(Turgut M)及巴蒂雷尔(Batirel)等人报告了脊柱结核病死率达 2%。在他们的研究中,694 例入组患者中有 314 例脊柱结核患者[27,31]。据报道,有 1/4 的患者因延误诊断而出现永久性后遗症。最常见的后遗症(4%~11%)是脊柱后凸/gibbus 畸形、脊柱侧凸、瘫痪、截瘫和感觉丧失[27]。高龄、脊柱畸形和神经功能障碍被认为是不良结局的预测因子[27]。

参考文献

[1] Trecarichi EM, Di Meco E, Mazzotta V, Fantoni M. Tuberculous spondylodiscitis: epidemiology, clinical features, treatment, and outcome. Eur Rev Med Pharmacol Sci. 2012; 16(Suppl 2): 58-72.
[2] Neumann JL, Schlueter DP. Retropharyngeal abscess as the presenting feature of tuberculosis of the cervical spine. Am Rev Respir Dis. 1974; 110: 508-511.
[3] Fang HS, Ong GB, Hodgson AR. Anterior spinal fusion: the operative approaches. Clin Orthop Relat Res. 1964; 35: 16-33.
[4] Peto HM, Pratt RH, Harrington TA, LoBue PA, Armstrong LR. Epidemiology of extrapulmonary tuberculosis in the United States, 1993-2006. Clin Infect Dis. 2009; 49: 1350-1357.
[5] Sharma SK, Mohan A. Extrapulmonary tuberculosis. Indian J Med Res. 2004; 120: 316-353.
[6] Pertuiset E, Beaudreuil J, Horusitzky A, et al. Epidemiological aspects of osteoarticular tuberculosis in adults. Retrospective study of 206 cases diagnosed in the Paris area from 1980 to 1994. Presse Med. 1997; 26: 311-315.
[7] Leonard MK, Blumberg HM. Musculoskeletal Tuberculosis. Microbiol Spectr. 2017; 5.
[8] Davidson PT, Horowitz I. Skeletal tuberculosis. A review with patient presentations and discussion. Am J Med. 1970; 48: 77-84.
[9] Agarwal RP, Mohan N, Garg RK, Bajpai SK, Verma SK, Mohindra Y. Clinicosocial aspect of osteo-articular tuberculosis. J Indian Med Assoc. 1990; 88: 307-309.
[10] Wang Y, Wang Q, Zhu R, et al. Trends of spinal tuberculosis research (1994-2015): a bibliometric study. Medicine (Baltimore). 2016; 95: e4923.
[11] Rauf F, Chaudhry UR, Atif M, ur Rahaman M. Spinal tuberculosis: our experience and a review of imaging methods. Neuroradiol J. 2015; 28: 498-503.
[12] Fuentes Ferrer M, Gutierrez Torres L, Ayala Ramirez O, Rumayor Zarzuelo M, del Prado Gonzalez N. Tuberculosis of the spine. A systematic review of case series. Int Orthop. 2012; 36: 221-231.

[13] De la Garza RR, Goodwin CR, Abu-Bonsrah N, et al. The epidemiology of spinal tuberculosis in the United States: an analysis of 2002 - 2011 data. J Neurosurg Spine. 2017; 26: 507 - 512.

[14] Leibert E, Schluger NW, Bonk S, Rom WN. Spinal tuberculosis in patients with human immunodeficiency virus infection: clinical presentation, therapy and outcome. Tuber Lung Dis. 1996; 77: 329 - 334.

[15] Donoghue HD, Lee OY, Minnikin DE, Besra GS, Taylor JH, Spigelman M. Tuberculosis in Dr Granville's mummy: a molecular re-examination of the earliest known Egyptian mummy to be scientifically examined and given a medical diagnosis. Proc Biol Sci. 2010; 277: 51 - 56.

[16] Zink A, Haas CJ, Reischl U, Szeimies U, Nerlich AG. Molecular analysis of skeletal tuberculosis in an ancient Egyptian population. J Med Microbiol. 2001; 50: 355 - 366.

[17] Crubezy E, Ludes B, Poveda JD, Clayton J, Crouau-Roy B, Montagnon D. Identification of Mycobacterium DNA in an Egyptian Pott's disease of 5,400 years old. C R Acad Sci III. 1998; 321: 941 - 951.

[18] Ratnappuli A, Collinson S, Gaspar-Garcia E, Richardson L, Bernard J, Macallan D. Pott's disease in twenty-first century London: spinal tuberculosis as a continuing cause of morbidity and mortality. Int J Tuberc Lung Dis. 2015; 19: 1125, i - ii.

[19] Ellner JJ. Review: the immune response in human tuberculosis — implications for tuberculosis control. J Infect Dis. 1997; 176: 1351 - 1359.

[20] Yadla M, Sriramnaveen P, Kishore CK, et al. Backache in patients on maintenance hemodialysis: beware of spinal tuberculosis. Saudi J Kidney Dis Transpl. 2015; 26: 1015 - 1017.

[21] Jevtic V. Vertebral infection. Eur Radiol. 2004; 14(Suppl 3): E43 - 52.

[22] Kaufmann SH, Cole ST, Mizrahi V, Rubin E, Nathan C. Mycobacterium tuberculosis and the host response. J Exp Med. 2005; 201: 1693 - 1697.

[23] De Vuyst D, Vanhoenacker F, Gielen J, Bernaerts A, De Schepper AM. Imaging features of musculoskeletal tuberculosis. Eur Radiol. 2003; 13: 1809 - 1819.

[24] Calderone RR, Larsen JM. Overview and classification of spinal infections. Orthop Clin North Am. 1996; 27: 1 - 8.

[25] Watts HG, Lifeso RM. Tuberculosis of bones and joints. J Bone Joint Surg Am. 1996; 78: 288 - 298.

[26] Shi T, Zhang Z, Dai F, et al. Retrospective study of 967 patients with spinal tuberculosis. Orthopedics. 2016; 39: e838 - 843.

[27] Batirel A, Erdem H, Sengoz G, et al. The course of spinal tuberculosis (Pott disease): results of the multinational, multicentre Backbone - 2 study. Clin Microbiol Infect. 2015; 21: 1008 e9 - e18.

[28] Pertuiset E, Beaudreuil J, Liote F, et al. Spinal tuberculosis in adults. A study of 103 cases in a developed country, 1980 - 1994. Medicine (Baltimore). 1999; 78: 309 - 320.

[29] Pigrau-Serrallach C, Rodriguez-Pardo D. Bone and joint tuberculosis. Eur Spine J. 2013; 22(Suppl 4): 556 - 566.

[30] Wang H, Yang X, Shi Y, et al. Early predictive factors for lower-extremity motor or sensory deficits and surgical results of patients with spinal tuberculosis: a retrospective study of 329 patients. Medicine (Baltimore). 2016; 95: e4523.

[31] Turgut M. Spinal tuberculosis (Pott's disease): its clinical presentation, surgical management, and outcome. A survey study on 694 patients. Neurosurg Rev. 2001; 24: 8 – 13.

[32] Wang LN, Wang L, Liu LM, Song YM, Li Y, Liu H. Atypical spinal tuberculosis involved noncontiguous multiple segments: case series report with literature review. Medicine (Baltimore). 2017; 96: e6559.

[33] Nigam A, Prakash A, Pathak P, Abbey P. Bilateral psoas abscess during pregnancy presenting as an acute abdomen: atypical presentation. BMJ Case Rep. 2013; 2013.

[34] Naim Ur R, El-Bakry A, Jamjoom A, Jamjoom ZA, Kolawole TM. Atypical forms of spinal tuberculosis: case report and review of the literature. Surg Neurol. 1999; 51: 602 – 607.

[35] Sharma A, Chhabra HS, Chabra T, Mahajan R, Batra S, Sangondimath G. Demographics of tuberculosis of spine and factors affecting neurological improvement in patients suffering from tuberculosis of spine: a retrospective analysis of 312 cases. Spinal Cord. 2017; 55: 59 – 63.

[36] Izawa K, Kitada S. Clinical analysis of Osteoarticular nontuberculous mycobacterial infection. Kekkaku. 2016; 91: 1 – 8.

[37] Kim CJ, Kim UJ, Kim HB, et al. Vertebral osteomyelitis caused by non-tuberculous mycobacteria: predisposing conditions and clinical characteristics of six cases and a review of 63 cases in the literature. Infect Dis (Lond). 2016; 48: 509 – 516.

[38] Deepti BS, Munireddy M, Kamath S, Chakrabarti D. Cervical spine tuberculosis and airway compromise. Can J Anaesth. 2016; 63: 768 – 769.

[39] Al SH. Retropharyngeal abscess associated with tuberculosis of the cervical spine. Tuber Lung Dis. 1996; 77: 563 – 565.

[40] El Azbaoui S, Alaoui Mrani N, Sabri A, et al. Pott's disease in Moroccan children: clinical features and investigation of the interleukin – 12/interferon-gamma pathway. Int J Tuberc Lung Dis. 2015; 19: 1455 – 1462.

[41] Nussbaum ES, Rockswold GL, Bergman TA, Erickson DL, Seljeskog EL. Spinal tuberculosis: a diagnostic and management challenge. J Neurosurg. 1995; 83: 243 – 247.

[42] Colmenero JD, Jimenez-Mejias ME, Sanchez-Lora FJ, et al. Pyogenic, tuberculous, and brucellar vertebral osteomyelitis: a descriptive and comparative study of 219 cases. Ann Rheum Dis. 1997; 56: 709 – 715.

[43] Kaila R, Malhi AM, Mahmood B, Saifuddin A. The incidence of multiple level noncontiguous vertebral tuberculosis detected using whole spine MRI. J Spinal Disord Tech. 2007; 20: 78 – 81.

[44] Polley P, Dunn R. Noncontiguous spinal tuberculosis: incidence and management. Eur Spine J. 2009; 18: 1096 – 1101.

[45] Yao DC, Sartoris DJ. Musculoskeletal tuberculosis. Radiol Clin N Am. 1995; 33:

679 - 689.
[46] Griffith JF, Kumta SM, Leung PC, Cheng JC, Chow LT, Metreweli C. Imaging of musculoskeletal tuberculosis: a new look at an old disease. Clin Orthop Relat Res. 2002; 398: 32 - 39.
[47] Raut AA, Naphade PS, Ramakantan R. Imaging Spectrum of Extrathoracic tuberculosis. Radiol Clin N Am. 2016; 54: 475 - 501.
[48] Jain R, Sawhney S, Berry M. Computed tomography of vertebral tuberculosis: patterns of bone destruction. Clin Radiol. 1993; 47: 196 - 199.
[49] Sharif HS, Morgan JL, al Shahed MS, al Thagafi MY. Role of CT and MR imaging in the management of tuberculous spondylitis. Radiol Clin N Am. 1995; 33: 787 - 804.
[50] Joo EJ, Yeom JS, Ha YE, et al. Diagnostic yield of computed tomography-guided bone biopsy and clinical outcomes of tuberculous and pyogenic spondylitis. Korean J Intern Med. 2016; 31: 762 - 771.
[51] Spira D, Germann T, Lehner B, et al. CT-guided biopsy in suspected spondylodiscitis — the Association of Paravertebral Inflammation with microbial pathogen detection. PLoS One. 2016; 11: e0146399.
[52] Ludwig B, Lazarus AA. Musculoskeletal tuberculosis. Dis Mon. 2007; 53: 39 - 45.
[53] Moore SL, Rafii M. Imaging of musculoskeletal and spinal tuberculosis. Radiol Clin N Am. 2001; 39: 329 - 342.
[54] Thammaroj J, Kitkuandee A, Sawanyawisuth K. Differences of Mri features between tuberculous and bacterial spondylitis in a Tb-endemic area. Southeast Asian J Trop Med Public Health. 2015; 46: 71 - 79.
[55] Jung NY, Jee WH, Ha KY, Park CK, Byun JY. Discrimination of tuberculous spondylitis from pyogenic spondylitis on MRI. AJR Am J Roentgenol. 2004; 182: 1405 - 1410.
[56] Phadke DM, Lucas DR, Madan S. Fine-needle aspiration biopsy of vertebral and intervertebral disc lesions: specimen adequacy, diagnostic utility, and pitfalls. Arch Pathol Lab Med. 2001; 125: 1463 - 1468.
[57] Colmenero JD, Ruiz-Mesa JD, Sanjuan-Jimenez R, Sobrino B, Morata P. Establishing the diagnosis of tuberculous vertebral osteomyelitis. Eur Spine J. 2013; 22(Suppl 4): 579 - 586.
[58] Merino P, Candel FJ, Gestoso I, Baos E, Picazo J. Microbiological diagnosis of spinal tuberculosis. Int Orthop. 2012; 36: 233 - 238.
[59] Lewinsohn DM, Leonard MK, Lobue PA, et al. Official American Thoracic Society/Infectious Diseases Society of America/Centers for Disease Control and Prevention clinical practice guidelines: diagnosis of tuberculosis in adults and children. Clin Infect Dis. 2017; 64: 111 - 115.
[60] Held M, Laubscher M, Mears S, et al. Diagnostic accuracy of the Xpert MTB/RIF assay for Extrapulmonary tuberculosis in children with musculoskeletal infections. Pediatr Infect Dis J. 2016; 35: 1165 - 1168.
[61] Held M, Laubscher M, Zar HJ, Dunn RN. GeneXpert polymerase chain reaction for spinal tuberculosis: an accurate and rapid diagnostic test. Bone Joint J. 2014; 96 - B: 1366 - 1369.

[62] Suzana S, Ninan MM, Gowri M, Venkatesh K, Rupali P, Michael JS. Xpert MTB/Rif for the diagnosis of extrapulmonary tuberculosis — an experience from a tertiary care Centre in South India. Tropical Med Int Health. 2016; 21: 385-392.

[63] Tali ET. Spinal infections. Eur J Radiol. 2004; 50: 120-133.

[64] Murray MR, Schroeder GD, Hsu WK. Granulomatous vertebral osteomyelitis: an update. J Am Acad Orthop Surg. 2015; 23: 529-538.

[65] Erdem H, Elaldi N, Batirel A, et al. Comparison of brucellar and tuberculous spondylodiscitis patients: results of the multicenter "Backbone-1 study". Spine J. 2015; 15: 2509-2517.

[66] Ye M, Huang J, Wang J, et al. Multifocal musculoskeletal tuberculosis mimicking multiple bone metastases: a case report. BMC Infect Dis. 2016; 16: 34.

[67] Nahid P, Dorman SE, Alipanah N, et al. Official American Thoracic Society/Centers for Disease Control and Prevention/Infectious Diseases Society of America clinical practice guidelines: treatment of drug-susceptible tuberculosis. Clin Infect Dis. 2016; 63: e147-e195.

[68] Moon MS. Tuberculosis of the spine. Controversies and a new challenge. Spine (Phila Pa 1976). 1997; 22: 1791-1797.

[69] Jain AK, Kumar S, Tuli SM. Tuberculosis of spine (C1 to D4). Spinal Cord. 1999; 37: 362-369.

[70] Fang D, Leong JC, Fang HS. Tuberculosis of the upper cervical spine. J Bone Joint Surg Br. 1983; 65: 47-50.

[71] Hsu LC, Leong JC. Tuberculosis of the lower cervical spine (C2 to C7). A report on 40 cases. J Bone Joint Surg Br. 1984; 66: 1-5.

[72] Pattisson PR. Pott's paraplegia: an account of the treatment of 89 consecutive patients. Paraplegia. 1986; 24: 77-91.

[73] Upadhyay SS, Saji MJ, Yau AC. Duration of antituberculosis chemotherapy in conjunction with radical surgery in the management of spinal tuberculosis. Spine (Phila Pa 1976). 1996; 21: 1898-1903.

[74] Ramachandran S, Clifton IJ, Collyns TA, Watson JP, Pearson SB. The treatment of spinal tuberculosis: a retrospective study. Int J Tuberc Lung Dis. 2005; 9: 541-544.

[75] Wang Z, Shi J, Geng G, Qiu H. Ultra-short-course chemotherapy for spinal tuberculosis: five years of observation. Eur Spine J. 2013; 22: 274-281.

[76] Blumberg HM, Leonard MK Jr, Jasmer RM. Update on the treatment of tuberculosis and latent tuberculosis infection. JAMA. 2005; 293: 2776-2784.

[77] Suarez-Garcia I, Noguerado A. Drug treatment of multidrug-resistant osteoarticular tuberculosis: a systematic literature review. Int J Infect Dis. 2012; 16: e774-778.

[78] Konstam PG, Blesovsky A. The ambulant treatment of spinal tuberculosis. Br J Surg. 1962; 50: 26-38.

[79] Jutte PC, van Loenhout-Rooyackers JH. Routine surgery in addition to chemotherapy for treating spinal tuberculosis. Cochrane Database Syst Rev. 2006: CD004532.

[80] Stratton A, Gustafson K, Thomas K, James MT. Incidence and risk factors for failed medical management of spinal epidural abscess: a systematic review and

meta-analysis. J Neurosurg Spine. 2017; 26: 81-89.
[81] Colmenero JD, Jimenez-Mejias ME, Reguera JM, et al. Tuberculous vertebral osteomyelitis in the new millennium: still a diagnostic and therapeutic challenge. Eur J Clin Microbiol Infect Dis. 2004; 23: 477-483.
[82] Nene A, Bhojraj S. Results of nonsurgical treatment of thoracic spinal tuberculosis in adults. Spine J. 2005; 5: 79-84.
[83] Khoo LT, Mikawa K, Fessler RG. A surgical revisitation of Pott distemper of the spine. Spine J. 2003; 3: 130-145.
[84] Kim YT, Han KN, Kang CH, Sung SW, Kim JH. Complete resection is mandatory for tubercular cold abscess of the chest wall. Ann Thorac Surg. 2008; 85: 273-277.
[85] Upadhyay SS, Sell P, Saji MJ, Sell B, Hsu LC. Surgical management of spinal tuberculosis in adults. Hong Kong operation compared with debridement surgery for short and long term outcome of deformity. Clin Orthop Relat Res. 1994: 173-182.
[86] Lifeso RM, Weaver P, Harder EH. Tuberculous spondylitis in adults. J Bone Joint Surg Am. 1985; 67: 1405-1413.
[87] Wang LJ, Zhang HQ, Tang MX, Gao QL, Zhou ZH, Yin XH. Comparison of three surgical approaches for thoracic spinal tuberculosis in adult: minimum 5-year follow up. Spine (Phila Pa 1976). 2017; 42: 808-817.
[88] Wang ST, Ma HL, Lin CP, et al. Anterior debridement may not be necessary in the treatment of tuberculous spondylitis of the thoracic and lumbar spine in adults: a retrospective study. Bone Joint J. 2016; 98-B: 834-839.
[89] Alam MS, Phan K, Karim R, et al. Surgery for spinal tuberculosis: a multi-center experience of 582 cases. J Spine Surg. 2015; 1: 65-71.
[90] Hodgson AR, Stock FE, Fang HS, Ong GB. Anterior spinal fusion. The operative approach and pathological findings in 412 patients with Pott's disease of the spine. Br J Surg. 1960; 48: 172-178.
[91] Garg N, Vohra R. Minimally invasive surgical approaches in the management of tuberculosis of the thoracic and lumbar spine. Clin Orthop Relat Res. 2014; 472: 1855-1867.
[92] Yang H, Hou K, Zhang L, et al. Minimally invasive surgery through the interlaminar approach in the treatment of spinal tuberculosis: a retrospective study of 31 patients. J Clin Neurosci. 2016; 32: 9-13.
[93] Oguz E, Sehirlioglu A, Altinmakas M, et al. A new classification and guide for surgical treatment of spinal tuberculosis. Int Orthop. 2008; 32: 127-133.
[94] Zhang X, Ji J, Liu B. Management of spinal tuberculosis: a systematic review and meta-analysis. J Int Med Res. 2013; 41: 1395-1407.
[95] Kumar K. Spinal tuberculosis, natural history of disease, classifications and principles of management with historical perspective. Eur J Orthop Surg Traumatol. 2016; 26: 551-558.
[96] Shelburne SA 3rd, Hamill RJ, Rodriguez-Barradas MC, et al. Immune reconstitution inflammatory syndrome: emergence of a unique syndrome during highly active antiretroviral therapy. Medicine (Baltimore). 2002; 81: 213-227.
[97] Shelburne SA, Montes M, Hamill RJ. Immune reconstitution inflammatory syndrome: more answers, more questions. J Antimicrob Chemother. 2006; 57: 167-170.

[98] Tang MX, Zhang HQ, Wang YX, Guo CF, Liu JY. Treatment of spinal tuberculosis by debridement, interbody fusion and internal fixation via posterior approach only. Orthop Surg. 2016; 8: 89-93.

[99] Cui X, Li LT, Ma YZ. Anterior and posterior instrumentation with different debridement and grafting procedures for multi-level contiguous thoracic spinal tuberculosis. Orthop Surg. 2016; 8: 454-461.

[100] Hassan K, Elmorshidy E. Anterior versus posterior approach in surgical treatment of tuberculous spondylodiscitis of thoracic and lumbar spine. Eur Spine J. 2016; 25: 1056-1063.

[101] Ran B, Xie YL, Yan L, Cai L. One-stage surgical treatment for thoracic and lumbar spinal tuberculosis by transpedicular fixation, debridement, and combined interbody and posterior fusion via a posterior-only approach. J Huazhong Univ Sci Technolog Med Sci. 2016; 36: 541-547.

[102] Zhang P, Peng W, Wang X, et al. Minimum 5-year follow-up outcomes for single-stage transpedicular debridement, posterior instrumentation and fusion in the management of thoracic and thoracolumbar spinal tuberculosis in adults. Br J Neurosurg. 2016; 30: 666-671.

[103] Gao Y, Ou Y, Deng Q, He B, Du X, Li J. Comparison between titanium mesh and autogenous iliac bone graft to restore vertebral height through posterior approach for the treatment of thoracic and lumbar spinal tuberculosis. PLoS One. 2017; 12: e0175567.

[104] Liu JM, Zhou Y, Peng AF, et al. One-stage posterior surgical management of lumbosacral spinal tuberculosis with nonstructural autograft. Clin Neurol Neurosurg. 2017; 153: 67-72.

[105] Jain A, Jain R, Kiyawat V. Evaluation of outcome of posterior decompression and instrumented fusion in lumbar and lumbosacral tuberculosis. Clin Orthop Surg. 2016; 8: 268-273.

[106] Sudprasert W, Piyapromdee U, Lewsirirat S. Neurological recovery determined by C-reactive protein, erythrocyte sedimentation rate and two different posterior decompressive surgical procedures: a retrospective clinical study of patients with spinal tuberculosis. J Med Assoc Thail. 2015; 98: 993-1000.

[107] Boxer DI, Pratt C, Hine AL, McNicol M. Radiological features during and following treatment of spinal tuberculosis. Br J Radiol. 1992; 65: 476-479.

[108] Kalita J, Misra UK, Mandal SK, Srivastava M. Prognosis of conservatively treated patients with Pott's paraplegia: logistic regression analysis. J Neurol Neurosurg Psychiatry. 2005; 76: 866-868.

8
结核性脑膜炎

德里亚·奥斯杜克-恩金和科尔内留·彼得鲁·波佩斯库

8.1 引言

结核性脑膜炎(tuberculous meningitis，TBM)是由结核分枝杆菌引起的重要公共卫生问题。中枢神经系统(central nervous system，CNS)结核占所有结核病例的1%，占EPTB病例的5%～10%[11]。结核病最具有破坏性的形式是结核性脑膜炎[7]。大约一半接受抗结核治疗的结核性脑膜炎患者会出现严重的后遗症或死亡[106]。TBM的神经系统后遗症包括颅神经麻痹、偏瘫/局灶性无力、认知障碍、运动障碍、视力障碍、中风、癫痫发作、听力障碍和意识改变[12,47,53,69]。

结核性脑膜炎的临床表现是非特异性的，并且用于诊断的实验室测试的敏感性低或需要很长时间，导致诊断延迟。延迟诊断和治疗对预后有不利影响[7,41]。

8.2 历史

分枝杆菌属被认为在数百万年前已经出现[21]。关于结核性脑膜炎的历史鉴定和引入，罗伯特·怀特(Robert Whytt)在1768年发表的一份报告中率先提出了临床体征和症状[8]。结核性脑膜炎最初被定义为独特的病理实体，并于1836年创造了"结核性脑膜炎"一词。这一定义是他将临床发现与死于急性脑积水的儿童的病理学观察联系起来的结果。他指出，结核病脑膜炎与结核病的相似之处，得出的结论是脑积水与肉芽组织和结核性浸润有关[109]。

接下来罗伯特·科赫(Robert Koch)在1882年发现并分离出结核病的

病原体[89]。詹姆斯·伦纳德·康宁(James Leonard Corning)于1885年率先进行了脊髓液的检查,而腰椎穿刺的发现归功于海因里希·昆克(Heinrich Quincke),后者也将其用于诊断目的,并于1891年将其用于临床[14,113]。里奇(Rich)和麦科多克(McCordock)进行了一系列的尸检,几乎在大多数TBM病例中记录了脑实质和脑膜中的干酪样区域。这些干酪样灶的破裂使细菌散布,使细菌进入蛛网膜下腔,引起脑膜炎[4,86]。

8.3 流行病学

据调查,全球约有1/3的人口患有隐性肺结核[52]。结核病是全球死亡的第九个原因。2016年,结核病病例为1 040万。值得注意的是,HIV感染者占所有结核病例的10%。有5个国家的结核感染人数占总人口的56%,包括印度、印度尼西亚、中国、菲律宾和巴基斯坦[77]。2014年,美国报告了9 412例新的结核病病例。病例总数(外国出生者的比率)是美国出生者的比率的13.4倍[94]。仅在2013年,土耳其共通报了13 409例病例,包括4 731例EPTB[49] (http://tuberkuloz.thsk.saglik.gov.tr/Dosya/Dokumanlar/raporlar/)。

在结核病高发国家,中枢神经系统结核通常困扰着年幼的儿童(<3岁),而在HIV低发国家中,大多数患者是移民成年人,他们是从结核病的高患病率国家移民而来的[103]。

HIV感染者患结核性脑膜炎的风险增加[119]。除HIV感染外,还报告了其他结核病危险因素,如糖尿病、营养不良、酒精中毒、恶性肿瘤以及使用免疫抑制剂[59,86]。大约75%的TBM患者与活动性结核病患者或有结核病史的人密切接触[56]。

卡介苗疫苗抗结核的保护尚有争议[102],据报道其对肺结核的保护作用欠佳。在随机对照试验中发现它可以预防粟粒型结核或结核性脑膜炎的发生率为86%,在病例对照研究中发现的预防率为75%[66,87]。

根据荟萃分析发现,卡介苗疫苗可提供50%的结核病防护[20],其他荟萃分析表明,卡介苗接种可预防结核病长达10年[1]。

8.4 病因及病理

结核分枝杆菌是一种革兰阳性细菌,由于其厚厚的细胞壁含有脂质、肽聚糖和阿拉伯甘露聚糖，所以染色较弱。仅与人相关的芽孢杆菌是专性好氧、无芽孢和抗酸的芽孢杆菌（acid-fast bacillus，AFB）。使用 Ziehl-Neelsen、Kinyoun 或金胺-罗丹明染料的标准染色技术可以检测到近 100 AFB/ml 的脑脊液[86]。与其他分裂时间为分钟的细菌相比，结核分枝杆菌的分裂极其缓慢，每 15～20 h 分裂 1 次。

结核分枝杆菌通过空气传播，吸入进入宿主体内。芽孢杆菌到达肺泡内的巨噬细胞并进行复制（图 8-1）[4]。原发复合征是肺部局部感染扩散到区域淋巴结。在这个阶段，会出现短暂但明显的菌血症，使结核杆菌可以扩散到身体的其他器官，包括脑膜或脑实质[7]。

在原发感染或播散性疾病后的菌血症期间，转移性干酪样病灶扩散到室管膜下或硬膜下结节（也称为"富病灶"），体积增大并破裂进入蛛网膜下腔。导致 TBM[66]。针对富集灶的炎症反应以及从富集灶释放的杆菌和结核抗原导致脑内的一些病理变化[7]。一项对脑脊液细胞因子水平的研究发 TNF-α、sTNFR-75、sTNFR-55、IFN-γ 和 IL-10 水平显著升高[67]。炎性浸润阻塞脑脊液会导致脑积水。血管炎导致梗死的发生，进而导致神经损伤[4]。在感染结核分枝杆菌的人群中，通常在暴露后的 1～2 年内有 10% 发展为活动性疾病[26]。尽管暴露，但研究人员仍然不清楚为什么这种疾病不会在一些人身上发展为活动性结核。可能是多因素造成的[102]。暴露于结核分枝杆菌病的结果可能基于病原体谱系（北京基因型），对人类基因功能的影响包括干扰素 γ、溶质载体家族 11、成员 1（SLC11A1）、TIRAP/MAL、P2XA7、CCL2、SNP T597C TLR2 和 LTA4H[7,15]。

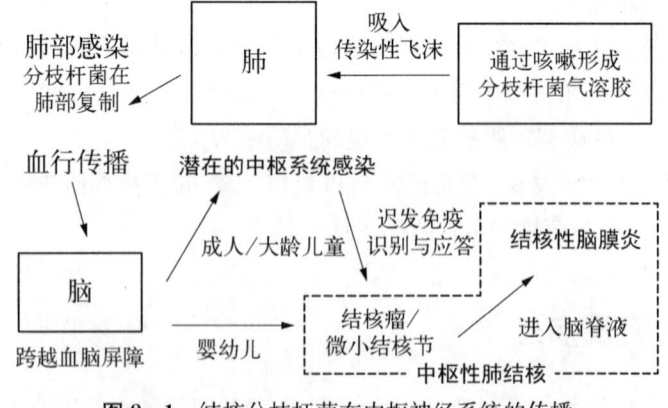

图 8-1　结核分枝杆菌在中枢神经系统的传播

8.5 病理学

除了脑膜，TBM 还会影响大脑的实质和血管系统。TBM 的组织病理学特征表现为厚厚的基底液，由淋巴细胞、单核细胞、上皮样组织细胞和坏死区组成，并伴有肉芽肿的形成。尸检研究记录了几乎所有病例(96%)的基底渗出物[17]。渗出物的形成可能阻碍脑脊液流动，导致脑积水；肉芽肿可能合并形成脓肿或结核球，导致局灶性神经功能缺损；闭塞性血管炎可能导致梗死和中风[109]。结核瘤的干酪性坏死中心被一个包膜包围，包膜内含有淋巴细胞、朗汉斯巨细胞、上皮样细胞和成纤维细胞[90]。

TBM 的血管受累范围包括动脉炎、动脉痉挛、动脉血栓形成和较大动脉被厚的渗出物压迫[17]。动脉炎经常影响大脑底部的主要动脉分支[72]。在急性暴发性病例中观察到坏死性病变，而在亚急性病例中更常见的是增生性病变[17]。

8.6 临床表现

TBM 的临床表现多种多样，包括慢性头痛或轻微的精神状态变化和普通脑膜炎的症状和体征，最常见的是头痛、发热、颈部僵硬、呕吐，严重的进行性脑膜炎会出现昏迷。前驱期出现不适、间歇性头痛、低热和体重减轻，在急性发作前 3～4 周，通常没有颈部强直[64,99]。在不同的研究中发热可能不一定出现，其中 19%～99% 的患者出现发热症状[3,58]。

在前驱期过后，随着脑膜炎症状的出现，TBM 的临床表现可能包括偏瘫、神志不清、癫痫发作、脑神经麻痹、运动障碍、复视、昏迷、运动障碍和昏迷[3]。有时，局灶性神经体征在没有前驱症状的情况下就会出现[64]。

根据患者年龄的不同，TBM 临床表现有所不同：儿童在前驱期出现咳嗽、发烧、呕吐(无腹泻)、身体不适和体重下降，而成人可能在 1～2 周内出现不适、体重减轻、低热和逐渐发作的头痛，随后头痛、呕吐和神志不清的情况恶化，如果不治疗会导致昏迷和死亡[107,108]。儿童头痛的发生率低于成人[86]。儿童最初也有更多的冷漠或易怒，意识水平下降，以及颅内压升高的迹象(通常是前囟门突出和外展神经麻痹)。另一方面，成年人有更多的脑神经麻痹(Ⅵ＞Ⅲ＞Ⅳ＞Ⅶ)，随着疾病的进展，意识模糊和昏迷加深；单瘫、偏瘫或截瘫[108]。

英国医学研究理事会(the British Medical Research Council，BMC)于1948年建立了结核性脑膜炎的严重程度分级，1974年随着格拉斯哥昏迷分级(Glasgow Coma Scale，GCS)的引入而完成。第一阶段(早期)相当于警觉和定向的无局灶性神经功能缺损的患者，GCS评分为15分。第二阶段(中期)首先对应患者的病情介于早期和晚期之间，但1974年后被定义为格拉斯哥昏迷评分11~14分或15分并有局灶性神经功能障碍。3级(晚期)相当于患者病情严重，处于深度昏迷状态，1974年后被定义为GCS小于或等于10分，并伴有或不伴有局灶性神经功能障碍[86,123]。

伴随脑膜外结核的临床表现可能出现，特别是肺部疾病；在其他病例中，没有临床或病史表现提示结核的病因[37,58]。在婴儿中，在TBM发生之前，首先发生原发肺部感染[108]。儿童结核性脑膜炎最常发生在原发结核病感染后3个月内[29]。

针对结核分枝杆菌的免疫应答影响着年轻患者(1岁以下)或HIV混合感染的患者[107,115]。在这些患者中，肺外扩散更容易，结核性脑膜炎可以突然发生，迅速演变为昏迷和虚弱，并与高病死率相关[123]。

在HIV混合感染的患者中，如果将TBM与隐球菌性脑膜炎进行比较，发现到TBM更常见症状的是颈项强直、发热和意识障碍[19]。TBM可导致严重的并发症：脑积水(80%的TBM患者有交通性脑积水)、结核球、脑室炎、血管炎和脑缺血,所有这些都导致TBM患者的高病死率和严重的后遗症。如果出现并发症，TBM的神经系统表现可能持续或恶化[123]。

8.7　诊断试验

常规实验室检查在TBM病例中不能得出特异性的结果，患者可能有白细胞减少、白细胞增多或白细胞计数正常[47,81]。TBM也可能与代谢并发症有关，最常见的是低钠血症，约有45%~79%的患者会出现低钠血症[23,70]。低钠血症可能源于脑性盐耗综合征、抗利尿激素分泌不当综合征、口渴感觉受损导致的过量液体摄入、甘露醇的使用或尿崩症的治疗[50]。

8.8 脑脊液分析

TBM 的诊断依赖于腰椎穿刺术后的脑脊液分析。脑脊液外观清晰或略呈乳白色。在 50% 的病例中，初始脑脊液压力超过 25 cmH$_2$O[109]。在室温或冰箱中保存时，脑脊液表面会形成类似蜘蛛网的外观[56]。TBM 患者的脑脊液中有中度的细胞增多症（表 8-1）。细胞计数为 100～500 cell/μl，以淋巴细胞为主，尽管在疾病的前 10 天可能有早期的多形核白细胞占优势[102]。据报道，在老年人和 HIV 感染者中也发现了无细胞脑脊液[16,54]。脑脊液蛋白水平在 100～500 mg/dl，血糖水平低于 45 mg/dl 或脑脊液/血浆比率低于 0.5 是典型的脑脊液病[66]。然而，有报道称脑脊液蛋白水平高于 5 g/L，血糖水平正常[117]。

表 8-1 合并结核性脑膜炎患者脑脊液检查

参考文献	例数	脑脊液葡萄糖 (mmol/L)	脑脊液蛋白 (mg/dl)	脑脊液白细胞 (/mm^3)
Verdon 等[117]a	47	1.9±1.3	345±286	273±722
Roca 等[85]b	29	1.33(0.94～1.77)	125(98～246)	148(65～388)
Hsu 等[48]a	46	2.35±1.90	346.3±548.1	221.8±306.5
He 等[44]a	161	2.11±1.53	138.7±70.4	198±198

a 平均值±标准差
b 中位数(最小值-最大值)

用 Erlich-Ziehl-Neelsen 染色检测脑脊液中的抗酸杆菌是一种廉价、快速的检测方法。它的灵敏度在 10%～60%，这取决于实验室和技术人员的经验[33]。通过增加显微镜检查的时间，大容量（10 ml）的脑脊液样本检查，以及重复的腰椎穿刺术可以提高检测的灵敏度[7,102]。脑脊液直接培养鉴定结核分枝杆菌是诊断的金标准。涂片镜检法和培养法分别需要 10^4～10^6 和 10^1～10^2 个细菌/毫升样本[6]。在 Lowenstein Jensen(L-J) 培养基上的培养阳性率在 25%～75%[7]。为了确保最大的敏感度，培养需要长达 8 周的时间，而且需要大量的劳动力。相反，在放射性液体培养基中培养可显著缩短持续时间，平均在 13 天即可得到阳性结果[51]。然而，在等待培养结果的同时尽早开始治疗是至关重要的。在 256 例结核分枝杆菌的研究中，放射性液体培养基和 L-J 培养基的分离率分别为 93% 和 39%[116]。在另一项研究中,自动培养和 L-J 系统的敏感率分别为 81.8% 和 72.7%。据报道,联合使用 L-J 和自动化系统比单独使用两种测试中的任何一种都要好[33]。

抗酸细菌涂片的低敏感性和获得培养结果的时间延长引发了对新诊断方法的探索。酶联免疫吸附试验用于检测脑脊液中针对特定分枝杆菌抗原的抗体。用间接酶联免疫吸附试验(ELISA)检测了 TBM 患者对 16 kDa 抗原的体液免疫应答(IgG 和 IgA),其敏感性为 42.8%,特异性为 94.7%[57]。

8.9 胸部 X 线片检查

在 30%～65% 的成年中枢神经系统结核患者中,胸部 X 线片检查显示出有活动性肺结核的表现[83,85,100]。在患有 TBM 的儿童中,HIV 感染者比非 HIV 感染者更有可能出现肺结核的 X 线片表现(84% : 70%)。与非 HIV 感染的患者相比,HIV 感染患者的肺门淋巴结病变、胸腔积液和空洞形成的发生率更高[100]。

8.10 放射学

计算机断层扫描(CT)和磁共振成像(MRI)提高结核性脑膜炎的诊断准确率。神经成像有助于早期诊断[46]。然而,30% 的患者有的脑 CT 扫描结果显示正常,大约 15% 的患者在结核性脑膜炎的早期阶段脑 MRI 扫描结果显示正常[2,123]。

结核性脑膜炎最常见的神经放射学特征包括基底性脑膜强化、脑积水以及幕上脑实质和脑干梗死[5]。结核性脑膜炎的出现是由于血行播散、富病灶破裂或脑脊液感染[22]直接延伸,在 CT 或 MRI 早期发现基底池有厚厚的胶状渗出物。最初,在疾病的早期阶段,平扫 MRI 检查通常很少或根本没有脑膜异常的证据,但随着疾病的发展,受影响的蛛网膜下腔肿胀,与正常脑脊液相比,T1 和 T2 松弛时间轻微缩短[111]。在大多数病例中,脑沟内、脑凸面和侧裂内的脑膜也有不同程度的受累。这些发现在钆增强磁共振成像中比在 CT 上更加明显[10]。通过对比增强 CT 成像确定的基底膜渗出物对 TBM 具有特异性,并预测不良预后[9]。脑膜在平扫 T1 加权磁化传递(MT)图像上表现为高信号,在增强后 T1 加权 MT 图像上进一步强化。

TBM 的 MT 比率明显高于病毒性脑膜炎,但低于真菌性或化脓性脑膜炎[39,43]。当 TBM 表现为视交叉蛛网膜炎时,会出现严重的视力丧失,基底液主要出现在脚间池、鞍上池和侧脑池,在 CT 扫描上呈"蜘蛛腿样"[40]。年龄和 HIV 混合感染会影响 TBM 的放射学特征;因此,TBM 儿童比 TBM 成人更容易出现脑积水。在同时感染 HIV-1 的人中,由于免疫反应受损导致基底性脑膜渗出物的缺乏,基底性增强通常不那么明显[24,55,123]。

脑膜强化的演变过程:尽管进行了适当的抗结核治疗,但脑膜强化最初仍有增加,在缺乏基础脑膜血管强化的情况下愈合,甚至在某些 TBM 病例中持续存在[5]。渗出物的扩展导致梗死和(或)出血,特别是在基底节和内囊区,这是 MRI 早期发现的[71]。在放射学上观察 TBM 的并发症对于确定治疗下的长期结果和演变是非常重要的。因此,MRI 对缺血和梗死的检测和定位增加了有关 TBM 演变的新数据[76,114]。用 MRI 检查小的软脑膜结核(约 90%的儿童和 70%的成人患有这种疾病)[108]和检测小范围的缺血或早期梗死比用 CT 扫描更可行[123]。

TBM 的一个罕见表现可能是颅内动脉瘤的形成[61,71]。结节性脑室炎在 MRI 上也是一种罕见的 TBM 并发症,在 MRI 的磁化传递图像上表现为室内间隔、脑室隔离和受影响脑室室管膜壁高信号[98]。

8.11 结核菌素皮肤试验

结核菌素皮肤试验(tuberculin skin test,TST)是用来确定一个人是否感染了结核分枝杆菌,感染后 2～8 周可检测到迟发性超敏反应。将 0.1 ml 5 TU 纯化蛋白衍生液注射到前臂皮内,在给药后 48～72 h 内读取和解释随后的反应,即可触摸到硬结的横径。对于免疫抑制的受试者,包括 HIV 感染者、与结核病病例有密切接触的人、有临床或放射学证据的当前或以前患有结核病的人,以及接受肿瘤坏死因子抑制剂治疗的个人,5 mm 硬结横径值或更大的硬化度被认为是阳性结果。对于潜伏性肺结核高危人群,例如出生在结核病高发国家或暴露于结核病职业风险中的人,硬结横径 10 mm 或以上的反应被认为是阳性。对于所有其他人,如果硬结横径大于或等于 15 mm,皮肤测试可能被认为是阳性[63]。

如果存在非结核分枝杆菌感染、测试用法错误、之前接种过卡介苗、阅读和解读错误,甚至使用了错误的抗原瓶,皮肤测试可能会产生假阳性结果。同样,假阴性结果可能与皮肤过敏、高龄(多年)或近期(暴露后 8～10 周内)的结核病感染、非常年轻(小于 6 个月)、某些病毒性疾病、最近接种活病毒疫苗(如麻疹或天花)、严重肺结核或对检测结果的不正确管理、阅读或解释[75]有关。

中枢神经系统结核患者中有 10%～50%的人皮肤试验呈阳性,而儿童的这一比率在 30%～65%[103]。

8.12 干扰素-γ释放试验(IGRAs)

干扰素-γ释放分析(IGRAs)是一种可用于诊断结核分枝杆菌感染的血液检测方法。然而,它们并不区分潜伏感染和结核病。Quantiferon®-TB Gold-in-Tube test(QFT-GIT)和 T-Spot®.TB test(T-SPOT test)是 FDA 批准的两种 IGRA 测试[63]。前者测量白细胞在面对 ESAT-6、CFP-10 和 TB7.7 等结核病特异性抗原时释放的干扰素-γ(IFN-g)浓度,后者测量 ESAT-6 和 CFP-10 激活的产生 IFN-g 的细胞数量[13,62]。据报道,测定干扰素-γ浓度的灵敏度为 90.2%[33]。在检测产生 IFNG 的细胞数量方面,特异性和敏感度分别为 92.8%和 83.6%[25]。皮试和 IGRAs 已在多项研究中进行了比较。一些人报告了类似的敏感率,而一些人报告说,与皮试相比,T-Spot 试验的敏感率更高,特别是在存在免疫抑制或粟粒型结核的情况下[60,68]。

8.13 结核硬脂酸

结核硬脂酸(tuberculostearic acid,TSA)是结核分枝杆菌的结构成分。在选择离子监测的情况下,使用气相色谱/质谱法在脑脊液中检测到它[38]。诊断为细菌性或病毒性脑膜炎的 6 例培养阳性患者中有 5 例阳性,19 例培养阴性患者中无阳性结果。在其他确诊实验室检测疑似 TBM 呈阴性的 10 例患者中,有 4 例患者采用这种方法获得了阳性结果[31]。

8.14 腺苷脱氨酶

腺苷脱氨酶(adenosine deaminase,ADA)是一种参与嘌呤分解代谢的酶,对单核细胞、巨噬细胞和T淋巴细胞的成熟起重要作用。它的活性在淋巴组织中升高,尤其是在活性T淋巴细胞中,这使其成为与T细胞介导的免疫反应相关疾病的重要标志物。该检测可用于TBM的确诊,但在其他中枢神经系统疾病如结节病、淋巴瘤并脑膜受累、蛛网膜下腔出血和神经布鲁菌病时,其活性也会增加[56]。

在一项涉及380名TBM患者的13项研究的荟萃分析中,评估了ADA试验在TBM诊断中的价值:1~4 U/L的水平有助于排除诊断(敏感性>93%,特异性<80%);4~8 U/L的水平不足以确认或排除诊断;高于8 U/L的水平被发现改善诊断(敏感性<59%,特异性>96%)[112]。脑脊液ADA活性对诊断有辅助作用,因此不推荐将其作为TBM的常规诊断试验[44]。

8.15　聚合酶链式反应(PCR)

结核杆菌培养周期的延长和对非培养诊断方法的需求增加,为基于分子方法检测脑脊液中的结核分枝杆菌铺平了道路。核酸扩增试验(nucleic acid amplification testing,NAAT)可以在临床标本或培养物中鉴定结核分枝杆菌。使用这种方法,甚至可以检测到少于10个细菌[109]。治疗开始后,脑脊液中可以检测到分枝杆菌DNA长达4周[30]。在对14项评估NAAT在TBM中价值的研究进行的荟萃分析中,该扩增试验显示敏感性为56%,特异性为98%[79]。涂阳呼吸道样本敏感度高,涂阳非呼吸道样本敏感度低。阴性结果并不排除结核病的诊断[109]。大多数基于PCR的研究可能会产生假阴性结果,这是因为在一些结核分枝杆菌分离株中使用了单一的靶基因进行扩增,并且缺少靶基因[66]。

聚合酶链式反应(polymerase chain reaction,PCR)是最常见的方法,但也有其他的扩增方法,如实时PCR、等温应变置换扩增、转录介导扩增和连接酶链式反应。WHO建议使用直线探针分析(line proke assays, LPAs)和Xpert MTB/RIF检测来检测结核分枝杆菌[109]。

8.16　治疗

TBM的治疗是迫在眉睫的。当临床高度怀疑TBM时,应立即开始抗结核治疗[73,120]。在获得细菌学证据之前,抗结核治疗不应拖延。病死率和发病率在很大程度上取决于治疗开始的阶段。平衡利弊是关键，延迟抗结核治疗（甚至只有几天）可能比在寻找正确诊断的同时进行不适当的治疗带来更大的危害。抗结核治疗包括两个基本环节：化疗和糖皮质激素。

对药物敏感的 TBM 的治疗遵循针对肺结核的治疗方案，即使这些建议没有考虑到抗结核药物很难穿透脑屏障，而且脑脊液中的浓度低于血浆水平的 10%~30%[28,32,45,74]。乙胺丁醇对脑膜疾病的疗效较差，甚至对存在炎症的脑膜的渗透性也很差[27]。WHO 建议所有患者服用 2 个月的利福平、异烟肼、吡嗪酰胺和乙胺丁醇，然后再服用 10 个月的利福平和异烟肼，但在 2003 年建议将乙胺丁醇改为链霉素[78]。然而，这两种药物（乙胺丁醇和链霉素）似乎都与患者的病情恶化有关，即使我们在疾病的早期就开始治疗[27]。

有关于最佳药物组合或治疗时间的随机对照试验。治疗从 4 种药物方案开始，为期 2 个月，然后继续两种药物方案（只有在分离株的敏感性可用的情况下），直到一年。治疗 TBM 的前三种抗菌药物包括异烟肼（INH）、利福平（RIF）和吡嗪酰胺（PZA），所有这些药物在有脑膜炎症的情况下都很容易进入脑脊液。利福平、异烟肼和吡嗪酰胺具有杀菌作用。口服制剂的生物可分解性使脑脊液水平超过敏感菌株所需的抑制浓度，因此这些药物可以口服。RIF 对这两种快速生长的生物亚群和半休眠生物都是有效的。INH 对快速生长的生物更为积极。PZA 具有良好的脑脊液穿透能力，对细胞内的分枝杆菌最有效。第四种药物可能是乙胺丁醇[73]、氟喹诺酮（莫西沙星或左氧氟沙星）或可注射氨基糖苷类药物（阿米卡星、卷曲霉素、卡那霉素或链霉素），只要脑膜炎症持续，每日给药共计 2 个月，因为氨基糖苷类药物只有在急性期才能渗透，超过此时间的作用尚不清楚[27]。氟喹诺酮类药物（莫西沙星或左氧氟沙星）在中枢神经系统中表现出良好的渗透性[27]。大剂量左氧氟沙星（每日 20 mg/kg）和利福平（每日 15 mg/kg）的强化治疗仍在争论中，研究表明，增加利福平剂量[88]和在标准方案中增加氟喹诺酮[104]可能会改善结核性脑膜炎和其他尚未证实有较高存活率患者的预后[45]。对于患有 TBM 的儿童，美国儿科学会（American Academy Of Pediatrics）建议，如果可能的话，最初的 4 种药物方案是异烟肼（INH）、RIF、PZA 和乙硫酰胺，或者前 2 个月使用氨基糖苷类药物[80]。治疗的持续时间需要逐个病例进行调整。对于结核球患者，疗程应延长至 18 个月。

二线药物是氟喹诺酮类药物（左氧氟沙星、莫西沙星、加替沙星）；注射用药氨基糖苷(阿米卡星、卷曲霉素、卡那霉素、链霉素);其他核心二线药物(乙硫酰胺/丙硫酰胺、环丝氨酸、利奈唑胺、氯法齐明),以及联合用药——不属于核心方案的药物(贝达奎兰、地拉曼、对氨基葡萄糖苷)。经验性二线治疗应在少数情况下开始:接触耐药结核病患者,在耐药结核病高发地区居住或旅行,以及治疗复发或治疗失败。

TBM 对利福平和异烟肼的多药耐药(multidrug resistance,MDR)导致病死率超过 80%[95,105,118]。对于耐多药结核病,目前还没有评价药物关联性或治疗时间的指南。WHO 建议使用至少 5 种有效药物(吡嗪酰胺和 4 种二线药物)的初始方案,并建议使用注射剂至少 8 个月[35]。MDR-TBM 的总疗程可能至少为 18 个月。及早和及时了解至少对异烟肼和 RIF 的耐药性将对设计抗结核疗法最有益[96]。在使用 GeneXpert MTB/RIF 的设置中,快速切换到二线药物可降低死亡率[123]。

在 HIV 合并感染和 TBM 中,早期开始抗逆转录病毒治疗可能会因免疫重建炎症综合征而复杂化。这可能表现为潜伏性结核病的重新激活,活动性结核病的进展,或者在以前抗结核治疗有所改善的患者中,表现为临床恶化。这就是为什么在未接受治疗的 HIV 合并结核性脑膜炎的患者中,无论 CD4 计数如何,抗逆转录病毒治疗的开始都应该从抗结核方案开始推迟 6~8 周[65,73,110]。另一方面,抗逆转录病毒治疗已被证明可以使 HIV 和 TBM 患者的 9 个月病死率降低到 40%以下[45]。

自 60 年前以来,颅内炎症和类固醇治疗的使用一直被认为是影响 TBM 预后的决定性因素[97]。一项对所有相关已发表试验的系统回顾和荟萃分析得出结论,皮质类固醇可提高 HIV-1 阴性儿童和成人 TBM 患者的存活率[82]。几种情况下急需激素治疗:化疗时或化疗前病情进展迅速的患者,表现为急性脑炎,脑脊液开放压力≥400 mmH$_2$O 或临床或 CT 表现为脑水肿的体征,抗结核化疗后临床体征"治疗矛盾"加剧,脑脊液蛋白>500 mg/dl 并升高(脊髓阻塞),CT 显示明显的基底动脉强化,以及中度或进展性脑积水或脑内结核[41,82,93,106]。结核瘤是 TBM 治疗的矛盾反应,即使没有对照试验,大剂量的辅助皮质类固醇也可用于治疗。皮质类固醇无效的结核性脑膜炎的其他辅助治疗方法可以是沙利度胺[92]。当其他辅助治疗(如皮质类固醇)无效时,可以使用沙利度胺。

血管炎和脑积水的出现可能是延迟治疗反应的原因[11]。TBM 合并脑积水的治疗可能需要脑室系统的手术减压,以有效控制颅内压升高的并发症。在等待化疗早期反应的同时,对于患有交通性脑积水的 2 期肺结核患者,联合使用连续腰椎穿刺术、皮质类固醇治疗和其他脱水剂(如乙酰唑胺、速尿和甘露醇)可能就足够了[84,91,121]。然而,对于昏迷患者,或者尽管接受了治疗,以进行性神经功能损害为特征的患者,手术过程不应延迟([84,42],GT)。对于非交通性脑积水,应采用脑室腹膜分流术(ventriculoperitoneal shunting, VPS)或内窥镜第三脑室造口术(endoscopic third ventriculostomy, ETV)进行手术干预[36]。与未感染 HIV 的患者相比,VPS 与 HIV 感染患者的预后更差[84]。与 ETV 相比,VPS 手术减压的适应证是困难的,也是尚未确定的。

8.17 预后

TBM 的病死率仍然高得令人无法接受,从 7%~69%[18,66]。研究表明多种因素影响 TBM 的预后,在一项对 507 例微生物学确诊的结核性脑膜炎患者的研究中,意识改变、糖尿病、免疫抑制、神经功能障碍、脑积水和血管炎对预后有不利影响。笔者开发了一种新的严重程度指数(Hamsi 评分),得分从 1 分到 6 分,得分最高的死亡率达到 40.1%[34]。

其他导致死亡的危险因素有:晚期或严重神经系统受累、昏迷、精神状态、延误诊断和治疗、癫痫发作、脑神经麻痹、极端年龄、异烟肼和利福平联合耐药、HIV 合并感染、CSF 参数如高 CSF 乳酸、CSF 白细胞减少、低 CSF 血糖和脑脊液培养阳性结核杆菌[47,48,66,86,101,122,123]。TBM 培养阳性与预后不良有关,这表明迅速减轻细菌负担可能是有益的。这些发现还表明,需要对结核性脑膜炎进行更具体的药动学和药效学研究。应用分子诊断方法的高质量研究可能为耐药结核性脑膜炎的治疗提供新的见解[123]。

参考文献

[1] Abubakar I, Pimpin L, Ariti C, Beynon R, Mangtani P, Sterne JA, Fine PE, Smith PG, Lipman M, Elliman D, Watson JM, Drumright LN, Whiting PF, Vynnycky E, Rodrigues LC. Systematic review and meta-analysis of the current evidence on the duration of protection by bacillus Calmette-Guerin vaccination against tuberculosis. Health Technol Assess. 2013; 17: 1-372, v-vi.
[2] Andronikou S, Smith B, Hatherhill M, Douis H, Wilmshurst J. Definitive neuroradiological diagnostic features of tuberculous meningitis in children. Pediatr

Radiol. 2004; 34: 876-885.
[3] Bang ND, Caws M, Truc TT, Duong TN, Dung NH, Ha DT, Thwaites GE, Heemskerk D, Tarning J, Merson L, Van Toi P, Farrar JJ, Wolbers M, Pouplin T, Day JN. Clinical presentations, diagnosis, mortality and prognostic markers of tuberculous meningitis in Vietnamese children: a prospective descriptive study. BMC Infect Dis. 2016; 16: 573.
[4] Be NA, Kim KS, Bishai WR, Jain SK. Pathogenesis of central nervous system tuberculosis. Curr Mol Med. 2009; 9: 94-99.
[5] Bernaerts A, Vanhoenacker FM, Parizel PM, Van Goethem JW, Van Altena R, Laridon A, De Roeck J, Coeman V, De Schepper AM. Tuberculosis of the central nervous system: overview of neuroradiological findings. Eur Radiol. 2003; 13: 1876-1890.
[6] Berwal A, Chawla K, Vishwanath S, Shenoy VP. Role of multiplex polymerase chain reaction in diagnosing tubercular meningitis. J Lab Physicians. 2017; 9: 145-147.
[7] Brancusi F, Farrar J, Heemskerk D. Tuberculous meningitis in adults: a review of a decade of developments focusing on prognostic factors for outcome. Future Microbiol. 2012; 7: 1101-1116.
[8] Breathnach CS. Robert Whytt (1714-1766): from dropsy in the brain to tuberculous meningitis. Ir J Med Sci. 2014; 183: 493-499.
[9] Bullock MR, Welchman JM. Diagnostic and prognostic features of tuberculous meningitis on CT scanning. J Neurol Neurosurg Psychiatry. 1982; 45: 1098-1101.
[10] Burrill J, Williams CJ, Bain G, Conder G, Hine AL, Misra RR. Tuberculosis: a radiologic review. Radiographics. 2007; 27: 1255-1273.
[11] Cag Y, Ozturk-Engin D, Gencer S, Hasbun R, Sengoz G, Crisan A, Ceran N, Savic B, Yasar K, Pehlivanoglu F, Kilicoglu G, Tireli H, Inal AS, Civljak R, Tekin R, Elaldi N, Ulu-Kilic A, Ozguler M, Namiduru M, Sunbul M, Sipahi OR, Dulovic O, Alabay S, Akbulut A, Sener A, Lakatos B, Andre K, Yemisen M, Oncu S, Nechifor M, Deveci O, Senbayrak S, Inan A, Dragovac G, Hc GL, Mert G, Oncul O, Kandemir B, Erol S, Agalar C, Erdem H. Hydrocephalus and vasculitis delay therapeutic responses in tuberculous meningitis: results of Haydarpasa-III study. Neurol India. 2016; 64: 896-905.
[12] Cagatay AA, Ozsut H, Gulec L, Kucukoglu S, Berk H, Ince N, Ertugrul B, Aksoz S, Akal D, Eraksoy H, Calangu S. Tuberculous meningitis in adults — experience from Turkey. Int J Clin Pract. 2004; 58: 469-473.
[13] Caglayan V, Ak O, Dabak G, Damadoglu E, Ketenci B, Ozdemir M, Ozer S, Saygý A. Comparison of tuberculin skin testing and QuantiFERON-TB Gold-In Tube test in health care workers. Tuberk Toraks. 2011; 59: 43-47.
[14] Calthorpe N. The history of spinal needles: getting to the point. Anaesthesia. 2004; 59: 1231-1241.
[15] Caws M, Thwaites G, Dunstan S, Hawn TR, Lan NT, Thuong NT, Stepniewska K, Huyen MN, Bang ND, Loc TH, Gagneux S, Van Soolingen D, Kremer K, Van Der Sande M, Small P, Anh PT, Chinh NT, Quy HT, Duyen NT, Tho DQ, Hieu NT, Torok E, Hien TT, Dung NH, Nhu NT, Duy PM, Van Vinh Chau N, Farrar J. The influence of host and bacterial genotype on the

development of disseminated disease with Mycobacterium tuberculosis. PLoS Pathog. 2008; 4: e1000034.
[16] Cecchini D, Ambrosioni J, Brezzo C, Corti M, Rybko A, Perez M, Poggi S, Ambroggi M. Tuberculous meningitis in HIV-infected and non-infected patients: comparison of cerebrospinal fluid findings. Int J Tuberc Lung Dis. 2009; 13: 269-271.
[17] Chatterjee D, Radotra BD, Vasishta RK, Sharma K. Vascular complications of tuberculous meningitis: An autopsy study. Neurol India. 2015; 63: 926-932.
[18] Christensen AS, Roed C, Omland LH, Andersen PH, Obel N, Andersen AB. Long-term mortality in patients with tuberculous meningitis: a Danish nationwide cohort study. PLoS One. 2011; 6: e27900.
[19] Cohen DB, Zijlstra EE, Mukaka M, Reiss M, Kamphambale S, Scholing M, Waitt PI, Neuhann F. Diagnosis of cryptococcal and tuberculous meningitis in a resource-limited African setting. Tropical Med Int Health. 2010; 15: 910-917.
[20] Colditz GA, Brewer TF, Berkey CS, Wilson ME, Burdick E, Fineberg HV, Mosteller F. Efficacy of BCG vaccine in the prevention of tuberculosis. Meta-analysis of the published literature. JAMA. 1994; 271: 698-702.
[21] Daniel TM. The history of tuberculosis. Respir Med. 2006; 100: 1862-1870.
[22] Dastur DK, Manghani DK, Udani PM. Pathology and pathogenetic mechanisms in neurotuberculosis. Radiol Clin N Am. 1995; 33: 733-752.
[23] Davis LE, Rastogi KR, Lambert LC, Skipper BJ. Tuberculous meningitis in the southwest United States: a community-based study. Neurology. 1993; 43: 1775-1778.
[24] Dekker G, Andronikou S, Van Toorn R, Scheepers S, Brandt A, Ackermann C. MRI findings in children with tuberculous meningitis: a comparison of HIV-infected and non-infected patients. Childs Nerv Syst. 2011; 27: 1943-1949.
[25] Di L, Li Y. The risk factor of false-negative and false-positive for T-SPOT.TB in active tuberculosis. J Clin Lab Anal. 2018; 32(2).
[26] Dinnes J, Deeks J, Kunst H, Gibson A, Cummins E, Waugh N, Drobniewski F, Lalvani A. A systematic review of rapid diagnostic tests for the detection of tuberculosis infection. Health Technol Assess. 2007; 11: 1-196.
[27] Donald PR. Cerebrospinal fluid concentrations of antituberculosis agents in adults and children. Tuberculosis (Edinb). 2010a; 90: 279-292.
[28] Donald PR. The chemotherapy of tuberculous meningitis in children and adults. Tuberculosis (Edinb). 2010b; 90: 375-392.
[29] Donald PR, Schaaf HS, Schoeman JF. Tuberculous meningitis and miliary tuberculosis: the Rich focus revisited. J Infect. 2005; 50: 193-195.
[30] Donald PR, Victor TC, Jordaan AM, Schoeman JF, Van Helden PD. Polymerase chain reaction in the diagnosis of tuberculous meningitis. Scand J Infect Dis. 1993; 25: 613-617.
[31] Elias J, De Coning JP, Vorster SA, Joubert HF. The rapid and sensitive diagnosis of tuberculous meningitis by the detection of tuberculostearic acid in cerebrospinal fluid using gas chromatography-mass spectrometry with selective ion monitoring. Clin Biochem. 1989; 22: 463-467.

[32] Ellard GA, Humphries MJ, Allen BW. Cerebrospinal fluid drug concentrations and the treatment of tuberculous meningitis. Am Rev Respir Dis. 1993; 148: 650-655.

[33] Erdem H, Ozturk-Engin D, Elaldi N, Gulsun S, Sengoz G, Crisan A, Johansen IS, Inan A, Nechifor M, Al-Mahdawi A, Civljak R, Ozguler M, Savic B, Ceran N, Cacopardo B, Inal AS, Namiduru M, Dayan S, Kayabas U, Parlak E, Khalifa A, Kursun E, Sipahi OR, Yemisen M, Akbulut A, Bitirgen M, Dulovic O, Kandemir B, Luca C, Parlak M, Stahl JP, Pehlivanoglu F, Simeon S, Ulu-Kilic A, Yasar K, Yilmaz G, Yilmaz E, Beovic B, Catroux M, Lakatos B, Sunbul M, Oncul O, Alabay S, Sahin-Horasan E, Kose S, Shehata G, Andre K, Alp A, Cosic G, Cem Gul H, Karakas A, Chadapaud S, Hansmann Y, Harxhi A, Kirova V, Masse-Chabredier I, Oncu S, Sener A, Tekin R, Deveci O, Karabay O, Agalar C. The microbiological diagnosis of tuberculous meningitis: results of Haydarpasa-1 study. Clin Microbiol Infect. 2014; 20: O600-608.

[34] Erdem H, Ozturk-Engin D, Tireli H, Kilicoglu G, Defres S, Gulsun S, Sengoz G, Crisan A, Johansen IS, Inan A, Nechifor M, Al-Mahdawi A, Civljak R, Ozguler M, Savic B, Ceran N, Cacopardo B, Inal AS, Namiduru M, Dayan S, Kayabas U, Parlak E, Khalifa A, Kursun E, Sipahi OR, Yemisen M, Akbulut A, Bitirgen M, Popovic N, Kandemir B, Luca C, Parlak M, Stahl JP, Pehlivanoglu F, Simeon S, Ulu-Kilic A, Yasar K, Yilmaz G, Yilmaz E, Beovic B, Catroux M, Lakatos B, Sunbul M, Oncul O, Alabay S, Sahin-Horasan E, Kose S, Shehata G, Andre K, Dragovac G, Gul HC, Karakas A, Chadapaud S, Hansmann Y, Harxhi A, Kirova V, Masse-Chabredier I, Oncu S, Sener A, Tekin R, Elaldi N, Deveci O, Ozkaya HD, Karabay O, Senbayrak S, Agalar C, Vahaboglu H. Hamsi scoring in the prediction of unfavorable outcomes from tuberculous meningitis: results of Haydarpasa-II study. J Neurol. 2015; 262: 890-898.

[35] Falzon D, Jaramillo E, Schunemann HJ, Arentz M, Bauer M, Bayona J, Blanc L, Caminero JA, Daley CL, Duncombe C, Fitzpatrick C, Gebhard A, Getahun H, Henkens M, Holtz TH, Keravec J, Keshavjee S, Khan AJ, Kulier R, Leimane V, Lienhardt C, Lu C, Mariandyshev A, Migliori GB, Mirzayev F, Mitnick CD, Nunn P, Nwagboniwe G, Oxlade O, Palmero D, Pavlinac P, Quelapio MI, Raviglione MC, Rich ML, Royce S, Rusch-Gerdes S, Salakaia A, Sarin R, Sculier D, Varaine F, Vitoria M, Walson JL, Wares F, Weyer K, White RA, Zignol M. WHO guidelines for the programmatic management of drug-resistant tuberculosis: 2011 update. Eur Respir J. 2011; 38: 516-528.

[36] Figaji AA, Fieggen AG, Peter JC. Endoscopic third ventriculostomy in tuberculous meningitis. Childs Nerv Syst. 2003; 19: 217-225.

[37] Fitzgerald Dw ST, Haas DW, Bennett EJ, Dolin R, Blaser MJ. Mycobacterium tuberculosis. In: Mandell, Douglas, and Bennett's principles and practice of infectious diseases, vol. 1. 8th ed. Philadelphia: Elsevier Churchill Livingstone; 2015. p. 2787-2818.

[38] French GL, Teoh R, Chan CY, Humphries MJ, Cheung SW, O'Mahony G. Diagnosis of tuberculous meningitis by detection of tuberculostearic acid in cerebrospinal fluid. Lancet. 1987; 2: 117-119.

[39] Gambhir S, Ravina M, Rangan K, Dixit M, Barai S, Bomanji J, International

Atomic Energy Agency Extra-Pulmonary, T. B. C. Imaging in extrapulmonary tuberculosis. Int J Infect Dis. 2017; 56: 237-247.

[40] Garg RK, Malhotra HS, Jain A. Neuroimaging in tuberculous meningitis. Neurol India. 2016; 64: 219-227.

[41] Girgis NI, Farid Z, Kilpatrick ME, Sultan Y, Mikhail IA. Dexamethasone adjunctive treatment for tuberculous meningitis. Pediatr Infect Dis J. 1991; 10: 179-183.

[42] GT, V. B. Complications in hydrocephalus shunting procedure. In: Wellenbur R, Brock M, Klinger M, editors. Advances in neurosurgery. 6th ed. New York: Springer; 1968. p. 28.

[43] Gupta RK, Kathuria MK, Pradhan S. Magnetization transfer MR imaging in CNS tuberculosis. AJNR Am J Neuroradiol. 1999; 20: 867-875.

[44] He Y, Han C, Chang KF, Wang MS, Huang TR. Total delay in treatment among tuberculous meningitis patients in China: a retrospective cohort study. BMC Infect Dis. 2017; 17: 341.

[45] Heemskerk AD, Bang ND, Mai NT, Chau TT, Phu NH, Loc PP, Chau NV, Hien TT, Dung NH, Lan NT, Lan NH, Lan NN, Phong Le T, Vien NN, Hien NQ, Yen NT, Ha DT, Day JN, Caws M, Merson L, Thinh TT, Wolbers M, Thwaites GE, Farrar JJ. Intensified antituberculosis therapy in adults with tuberculous meningitis. N Engl J Med. 2016; 374: 124-134.

[46] Hooijboer PG, Van Der Vliet AM, Sinnige LG. Tuberculous meningitis in native Dutch children: a report of four cases. Pediatr Radiol. 1996; 26: 542-546.

[47] Hosoglu S, Geyik MF, Balik I, Aygen B, Erol S, Aygencel TG, Mert A, Saltoglu N, Dokmetas I, Felek S, Sunbul M, Irmak H, Aydin K, Kokoglu OF, Ucmak H, Altindis M, Loeb M. Predictors of outcome in patients with tuberculous meningitis. Int J Tuberc Lung Dis. 2002; 6: 64-70.

[48] Hsu PC, Yang CC, Ye JJ, Huang PY, Chiang PC, Lee MH. Prognostic factors of tuberculous meningitis in adults: a 6-year retrospective study at a tertiary hospital in northern Taiwan. J Microbiol Immunol Infect. 2010; 43: 111-118.

[49] http://tuberkuloz.thsk.saglik.gov.tr/Dosya/Dokumanlar/raporlar/.turkiyede_verem_savasi_2015_raporu.pdf.

[50] Inamdar P, Masavkar S, Shanbag P. Hyponatremia in children with tuberculous meningitis: a hospital-based cohort study. J Pediatr Neurosci. 2016; 11: 182-187.

[51] Jonas V, Alden MJ, Curry JI, Kamisango K, Knott CA, Lankford R, Wolfe JM, Moore DF. Detection and identification of Mycobacterium tuberculosis directly from sputum sediments by amplification of rRNA. J Clin Microbiol. 1993; 31: 2410-2416.

[52] Jullien S, Ryan H, Modi M, Bhatia R. Six months therapy for tuberculous meningitis. Cochrane Database Syst Rev. 2016; 9: CD012091.

[53] Kalita J, Misra UK, Ranjan P. Predictors of long-term neurological sequelae of tuberculous meningitis: a multivariate analysis. Eur J Neurol. 2007; 14: 33-37.

[54] Karstaedt AS, Valtchanova S, Barriere R, Crewe-Brown HH. Tuberculous meningitis in South African urban adults. QJM. 1998; 91: 743-747.

[55] Katrak SM, Shembalkar PK, Bijwe SR, Bhandarkar LD. The clinical, radiological and pathological profile of tuberculous meningitis in patients with and

without human immunodeficiency virus infection. J Neurol Sci. 2000; 181: 118 - 126.
[56] Katti MK. Pathogenesis, diagnosis, treatment, and outcome aspects of cerebral tuberculosis. Med Sci Monit. 2004; 10: RA215 - 229.
[57] Kaushik A, Singh UB, Porwal C, Venugopal SJ, Mohan A, Krishnan A, Goyal V, Banavaliker JN. Diagnostic potential of 16 kDa (HspX, alpha-crystalline) antigen for serodiagnosis of tuberculosis. Indian J Med Res. 2012; 135: 771 - 777.
[58] Kennedy DH, Fallon RJ. Tuberculous meningitis. JAMA. 1979; 241: 264 - 268.
[59] Kumar NP, Babu S. Influence of diabetes mellitus on the immunity to human tuberculosis. Immunology. 2017; 152: 13.
[60] Lee YM, Park KH, Kim SM, Park SJ, Lee SO, Choi SH, Kim YS, Woo JH, Kim SH. Risk factors for false-negative results of T-SPOT.TB and tuberculin skin test in extrapulmonary tuberculosis. Infection. 2013; 41: 1089 - 1095.
[61] Leiguarda R, Berthier M, Starkstein S, Nogues M, Lylyk P. Ischemic infarction in 25 children with tuberculous meningitis. Stroke. 1988; 19: 200 - 204.
[62] Lempp JM, Zajdowicz MJ, Hankinson AL, Toney SR, Keep LW, Mancuso JD, Mazurek GH. Assessment of the QuantiFERON-TB Gold In-Tube test for the detection of Mycobacterium tuberculosis infection in United States Navy recruits. PLoS One. 2017; 12: e0177752.
[63] Lewinsohn DM, Leonard MK, Lobue PA, Cohn DL, Daley CL, Desmond E, Keane J, Lewinsohn DA, Loeffler AM, Mazurek GH, O'Brien RJ, Pai M, Richeldi L, Salfinger M, Shinnick TM, Sterling TR, Warshauer DM, Woods GL. Official American Thoracic Society/Infectious Diseases Society of America/Centers for disease control and prevention clinical practice guidelines: diagnosis of tuberculosis in adults and children. Clin Infect Dis. 2017; 64: e1 - e33.
[64] Lincoln EM, Sordillo VR, Davies PA. Tuberculous meningitis in children. A review of 167 untreated and 74 treated patients with special reference to early diagnosis. J Pediatr. 1960; 57: 807 - 823.
[65] Marais S, Meintjes G, Pepper DJ, Dodd LE, Schutz C, Ismail Z, Wilkinson KA, Wilkinson RJ. Frequency, severity, and prediction of tuberculous meningitis immune reconstitution inflammatory syndrome. Clin Infect Dis. 2013; 56: 450 - 460.
[66] Marx GE, Chan ED. Tuberculous meningitis: diagnosis and treatment overview. Tuberc Res Treat. 2011; 2011: 798764.
[67] Mastroianni CM, Paoletti F, Lichtner M, D'Agostino C, Vullo V, Delia S. Cerebrospinal fluid cytokines in patients with tuberculous meningitis. Clin Immunol Immunopathol. 1997; 84: 171 - 176.
[68] Mazurek GH, Weis SE, Moonan PK, Daley CL, Bernardo J, Lardizabal AA, Reves RR, Toney SR, Daniels LJ, Lobue PA. Prospective comparison of the tuberculin skin test and 2 whole-blood interferon-gamma release assays in persons with suspected tuberculosis. Clin Infect Dis. 2007; 45: 837 - 845.
[69] Merkler AE, Reynolds AS, Gialdini G, Morris NA, Murthy SB, Thakur K, Kamel H. Neurological complications after tuberculous meningitis in a multi-state cohort in the United States. J Neurol Sci. 2017; 375: 460 - 463.
[70] Misra UK, Kalita J, Bhoi SK, Singh RK. A study of hyponatremia in tuberculous meningitis. J Neurol Sci. 2016; 367: 152 - 157.

[71] Morgado C, Ruivo N. Imaging meningo-encephalic tuberculosis. Eur J Radiol. 2005; 55: 188-192.

[72] Murthy JM. Tuberculous meningitis: the challenges. Neurol India. 2010; 58: 716-722.

[73] Nahid P, Dorman SE, Alipanah N, Barry PM, Brozek JL, Cattamanchi A, Chaisson LH, Chaisson RE, Daley CL, Grzemska M, Higashi JM, Ho CS, Hopewell PC, Keshavjee SA, Lienhardt C, Menzies R, Merrifield C, Narita M, O'Brien R, Peloquin CA, Raftery A, Saukkonen J, Schaaf HS, Sotgiu G, Starke JR, Migliori GB, Vernon A. Official American Thoracic Society/Centers for Disease Control and Prevention/Infectious Diseases Society of America Clinical Practice Guidelines: treatment of drug-susceptible tuberculosis. Clin Infect Dis. 2016; 63: e147-195.

[74] Nau R, Prange HW, Menck S, Kolenda H, Visser K, Seydel JK. Penetration of rifampicin into the cerebrospinal fluid of adults with uninflamed meninges. J Antimicrob Chemother. 1992; 29: 719-724.

[75] Nayak S, Acharjya B. Mantoux test and its interpretation. Indian Dermatol Online J. 2012; 3: 2-6.

[76] Omar N, Andronikou S, Van Toorn R, Pienaar M. Diffusion-weighted magnetic resonance imaging of borderzone necrosis in paediatric tuberculous meningitis. J Med Imaging Radiat Oncol. 2011; 55: 563-570.

[77] ORGANIZATION 2017. WH. Global tuberculosis report.

[78] ORGANIZATION, W. H. 2003. Guidelines for the management of sexually transmitted infections, World Health Organization.

[79] Pai M, Flores LL, Pai N, Hubbard A, Riley LW, Colford JM Jr. Diagnostic accuracy of nucleic acid amplification tests for tuberculous meningitis: a systematic review and meta-analysis. Lancet Infect Dis. 2003; 3: 633-643.

[80] PEDIATRICS., A. A. O. Committee on infectious diseases. In: Red book: report of the committee on infectious diseases. 30th ed. Elk Grove Village: AAP; 2015. p. 2015.

[81] Pehlivanoglu F, Yasar KK, Sengoz G. Tuberculous meningitis in adults: a review of 160 cases. ScientificWorldJournal. 2012; 2012: 169028.

[82] Prasad K, Singh MB, Ryan H. Corticosteroids for managing tuberculous meningitis. Cochrane Database Syst Rev. 2016; 4: CD002244.

[83] Qureshi H, Merwat S, Nawaz S, Rana A, Malik A, Mahmud M, Latif A, Khan A, Sarwari A. Predictors of inpatient mortality in 190 adult patients with tuberculous meningitis. J Pak Med Assoc. 2002; 52: 159-163.

[84] Rizvi I, Garg RK, Malhotra HS, Kumar N, Sharma E, Srivastava C, Uniyal R. Ventriculo-peritoneal shunt surgery for tuberculous meningitis: a systematic review. J Neurol Sci. 2017; 375: 255-263.

[85] Roca B, Tornador N, Tornador E. Presentation and outcome of tuberculous meningitis in adults in the province of Castellon, Spain: a retrospective study. Epidemiol Infect. 2008; 136: 1455-1462.

[86] Rock RB, Olin M, Baker CA, Molitor TW, Peterson PK. Central nervous system tuberculosis: pathogenesis and clinical aspects. Clin Microbiol Rev. 2008; 21: 243-261. table of contents.

[87] Rodrigues LC, Diwan VK, Wheeler JG. Protective effect of BCG against tuberculous meningitis and miliary tuberculosis: a meta-analysis. Int J Epidemiol. 1993; 22: 1154-1158.

[88] Ruslami R, Ganiem AR, Dian S, Apriani L, Achmad TH, Van Der Ven AJ, Borm G, Aarnoutse RE, Van Crevel R. Intensified regimen containing rifampicin and moxifloxacin for tuberculous meningitis: an open-label, randomised controlled phase 2 trial. Lancet Infect Dis. 2013; 13: 27-35.

[89] Sakula A. Robert koch: centenary of the discovery of the tubercle bacillus, 1882. Can Vet J. 1983; 24: 127-131.

[90] Sanei Taheri M, Karimi MA, Haghighatkhah H, Pourghorban R, Samadian M, Delavar Kasmaei H. Central nervous system tuberculosis: an imaging-focused review of a reemerging disease. Radiol Res Pract. 2015; 2015: 202806.

[91] Schoeman J, Donald P, Van Zyl L, Keet M, Wait J. Tuberculous hydrocephalus: comparison of different treatments with regard to ICP, ventricular size and clinical outcome. Dev Med Child Neurol. 1991; 33: 396-405.

[92] Schoeman JF, Andronikou S, Stefan DC, Freeman N, Van Toorn R. Tuberculous meningitis-related optic neuritis: recovery of vision with thalidomide in 4 consecutive cases. J Child Neurol. 2010; 25: 822-828.

[93] Schoeman JF, Van Zyl LE, Laubscher JA, Donald PR. Effect of corticosteroids on intracranial pressure, computed tomographic findings, and clinical outcome in young children with tuberculous meningitis. Pediatrics. 1997; 99: 226-231.

[94] Scott C, Kirking HL, Jeffries C, Price SF, Pratt R, Centers for Disease, C. & Prevention. Tuberculosis trends — United States, 2014. MMWR Morb Mortal Wkly Rep. 2015; 64: 265-269.

[95] Seddon JA, Visser DH, Bartens M, Jordaan AM, Victor TC, Van Furth AM, Schoeman JF, Schaaf HS. Impact of drug resistance on clinical outcome in children with tuberculous meningitis. Pediatr Infect Dis J. 2012; 31: 711-716.

[96] Senbayrak S, Ozkutuk N, Erdem H, Johansen IS, Civljak R, Inal AS, Kayabas U, Kursun E, Elaldi N, Savic B, Simeon S, Yilmaz E, Dulovic O, Ozturk-Engin D, Ceran N, Lakatos B, Sipahi OR, Sunbul M, Yemisen M, Alabay S, Beovic B, Ulu-Kilic A, Cag Y, Catroux M, Inan A, Dragovac G, Deveci O, Tekin R, Gul HC, Sengoz G, Andre K, Harxhi A, Hansmann Y, Oncu S, Kose S, Oncul O, Parlak E, Sener A, Yilmaz G, Savasci U, Vahaboglu H. Antituberculosis drug resistance patterns in adults with tuberculous meningitis: results of haydarpasa-iv study. Ann Clin Microbiol Antimicrob. 2015; 14: 47.

[97] Shane SJ, Clowater RA, Riley C. The treatment of tuberculous meningitis with cortisone and streptomycin. Can Med Assoc J. 1952; 67: 13-15.

[98] Singh P, Paliwal VK, Neyaz Z, Srivastava AK, Verma R, Mohan S. Clinical and magnetic resonance imaging characteristics of tubercular ventriculitis: an under-recognized complication of tubercular meningitis. J Neurol Sci. 2014; 342: 137-140.

[99] Smith HV, Vollum RL. The diagnosis of tuberculous meningitis. Br Med Bull. 1954; 10: 140-145.

[100] Solomons RS, Goussard P, Visser DH, Marais BJ, Gie RP, Schoeman JF, Van

Furth AM. Chest radiograph findings in children with tuberculous meningitis. Int J Tuberc Lung Dis. 2015; 19: 200-204.

[101] Tan EK, Chee MW, Chan LL, Lee YL. Culture positive tuberculous meningitis: clinical indicators of poor prognosis. Clin Neurol Neurosurg. 1999; 101: 157-160.

[102] Thwaites G, Chau TT, Mai NT, Drobniewski F, McAdam K, Farrar J. Tuberculous meningitis. J Neurol Neurosurg Psychiatry. 2000; 68: 289-299.

[103] Thwaites G, Fisher M, Hemingway C, Scott G, Solomon T, Innes J, British Infection S. British Infection Society guidelines for the diagnosis and treatment of tuberculosis of the central nervous system in adults and children. J Infect. 2009; 59: 167-187.

[104] Thwaites GE, Bhavnani SM, Chau TT, Hammel JP, Torok ME, Van Wart SA, Mai PP, Reynolds DK, Caws M, Dung NT, Hien TT, Kulawy R, Farrar J, Ambrose PG. Randomized pharmacokinetic and pharmacodynamic comparison of fluoroquinolones for tuberculous meningitis. Antimicrob Agents Chemother. 2011; 55: 3244-3253.

[105] Thwaites GE, Lan NT, Dung NH, Quy HT, Oanh DT, Thoa NT, Hien NQ, Thuc NT, Hai NN, Bang ND, Lan NN, Duc NH, Tuan VN, Hiep CH, Chau TT, Mai PP, Dung NT, Stepniewska K, White NJ, Hien TT, Farrar JJ. Effect of antituberculosis drug resistance on response to treatment and outcome in adults with tuberculous meningitis. J Infect Dis. 2005; 192: 79-88.

[106] Thwaites GE, Nguyen DB, Nguyen HD, Hoang TQ, Do TT, Nguyen TC, Nguyen QH, Nguyen TT, Nguyen NH, Nguyen TN, Nguyen NL, Nguyen HD, Vu NT, Cao HH, Tran TH, Pham PM, Nguyen TD, Stepniewska K, White NJ, Tran TH, Farrar JJ. Dexamethasone for the treatment of tuberculous meningitis in adolescents and adults. N Engl J Med. 2004; 351: 1741-1751.

[107] Thwaites GE, Tran TH. Tuberculous meningitis: many questions, too few answers. Lancet Neurol. 2005; 4: 160-170.

[108] Thwaites GE, Van Toorn R, Schoeman J. Tuberculous meningitis: more questions, still too few answers. Lancet Neurol. 2013; 12: 999-1010.

[109] Torok ME. Tuberculous meningitis: advances in diagnosis and treatment. Br Med Bull. 2015; 113: 117-131.

[110] Torok ME, Yen NT, Chau TT, Mai NT, Phu NH, Mai PP, Dung NT, Chau NV, Bang ND, Tien NA, Minh NH, Hien NQ, Thai PV, Dong DT, Anh DT, Thoa NT, Hai NN, Lan NN, Lan NT, Quy HT, Dung NH, Hien TT, Chinh NT, Simmons CP, De Jong M, Wolbers M, Farrar JJ. Timing of initiation of antiretroviral therapy in human immunodeficiency virus (HIV)-associated tuberculous meningitis. Clin Infect Dis. 2011; 52: 1374-1383.

[111] Trivedi R, Saksena S, Gupta RK. Magnetic resonance imaging in central nervous system tuberculosis. Indian J Radiol Imaging. 2009; 19: 256-265.

[112] Tuon FF, Higashino HR, Lopes MI, Litvoc MN, Atomiya AN, Antonangelo L, Leite OM. Adenosine deaminase and tuberculous meningitis — a systematic review with meta-analysis. Scand J Infect Dis. 2010; 42: 198-207.

[113] Tyler KL. Chapter 28: a history of bacterial meningitis. Handb Clin Neurol. 2010; 95: 417-433.

[114] Van Der Merwe DJ, Andronikou S, Van Toorn R, Pienaar M. Brainstem ischemic lesions on MRI in children with tuberculous meningitis: with diffusion weighted confirmation. Childs Nerv Syst. 2009; 25: 949-954.

[115] Van Well GT, Paes BF, Terwee CB, Springer P, Roord JJ, Donald PR, Van Furth AM, Schoeman JF. Twenty years of pediatric tuberculous meningitis: a retrospective cohort study in the western cape of South Africa. Pediatrics. 2009; 123: e1-8.

[116] Venkataswamy MM, Rafi W, Nagarathna S, Ravi V, Chandramuki A. Comparative evaluation of BACTEC 460TB system and Lowenstein-Jensen medium for the isolation of M. tuberculosis from cerebrospinal fluid samples of tuberculous meningitis patients. Indian J Med Microbiol. 2007; 25: 236-240.

[117] Verdon R, Chevret S, Laissy JP, Wolff M. Tuberculous meningitis in adults: review of 48 cases. Clin Infect Dis. 1996; 22: 982-988.

[118] Vinnard C, King L, Munsiff S, Crossa A, Iwata K, Pasipanodya J, Proops D, Ahuja S. Long-term mortality of patients with tuberculous meningitis in New York City: a cohort study. Clin Infect Dis. 2017; 64: 401-407.

[119] Vinnard C, Macgregor RR. Tuberculous meningitis in HIV-infected individuals. Curr HIV/AIDS Rep. 2009; 6: 139-145.

[120] Vinnard C, Winston CA, Wileyto EP, Macgregor RR, Bisson GP. Isoniazid resistance and death in patients with tuberculous meningitis: retrospective cohort study. BMJ. 2010; 341: c4451.

[121] Visudhiphan P, Chiemchanya S. Hydrocephalus in tuberculous meningitis in children: treatment with acetazolamide and repeated lumbar puncture. J Pediatr. 1979; 95: 657-660.

[122] Wang JT, Hung CC, Sheng WH, Wang JY, Chang SC, Luh KT. Prognosis of tuberculous meningitis in adults in the era of modern antituberculous chemotherapy. J Microbiol Immunol Infect. 2002; 35: 215-222.

[123] Wilkinson RJ, Rohlwink U, Misra UK, Van Crevel R, Mai NTH, Dooley KE, Caws M, Figaji A, Savic R, Solomons R, Thwaites GE, Tuberculous Meningitis International Research, C. Tuberculous meningitis. Nat Rev Neurol. 2017; 13: 581-598.

[124] Yaramis A, Bukte Y, Katar S, Ozbek MN. Chest computerized tomography scan findings in 74 children with tuberculous meningitis in southeastern Turkey. Turk J Pediatr. 2007; 49: 365-369.

9
结核性脑炎

琼·保罗·斯塔尔

9.1 背景

结核病是一种多部位感染的疾病,最常见在肺部。从最初的感染开始,细菌通过血液在体内传播,产生菌血症的作用。感染性转移是多种多样的,其中以脑转移最为严重。

脑炎和脑膜炎很难区分,因为它们最常合并感染。可以说,中枢神经系统症状的重要性更倾向于脑炎而不是脑膜炎。为了方便在国际水平的研究之间进行比较,最近专家公布了结核性脑炎的定义[1]:

需要一个主要标准:患者应出现精神状态改变(定义为意识水平降低或改变、嗜睡或个人性格改变)持续≥24 h,没有发现其他原因;

需要较小的标准——可能的脑炎需要两个标准,可能或确诊的脑炎需要3个或更多的标准:

1. 在出院前或入院后72 h内记录的体温≥38℃(100.4℉);
2. 不完全归因于先前存在的癫痫障碍的全面性或部分癫痫发作;
3. 新的局灶性神经学发现;
4. 脑脊液白细胞计数≥5/mm^3;
5. 神经影像上的脑实质异常提示脑炎,要么是先前研究中的新发现,要么是发病时看起来很严重;
6. 脑电图异常,与脑炎相一致,不能归因于其他原因。

9.2 流行病学

从2003年到2014年,27个欧盟/欧洲经济区国家共报告了564 916例肺结核病例,其中83%表现为单纯肺部感染,17%表现为肺外疾病。据报道,3%的肺外感染涉及神经系统[2]。

在法国,一项约253例传染性脑炎[3]的研究报告了20例结核性脑炎病例(占所有病例的5%,占已确诊病例的15%),分类为确诊病例(60%)、拟诊病例(20%)和疑似病例(20%)。

难民危机使人口混杂在一起。从2004年到2013年,西班牙的一项研究报告说,在2426名移民中,撒哈拉以南地区2.85%的患者出现肺外结核,11%的患者来自马格里布,4.4%的患者来自东欧,1.5%的患者来自拉丁美洲[4]。

在两项欧洲研究中,一项在法国[5],另一项在英国[6],结核性脑炎似乎分别占有病因学诊断的脑炎的15%(占所有病例的8%,包括未确诊的病例)和显示的感染性脑炎的12%。在法国的研究中,最有可能先前已感染结核但最近临床发病的患者中,发现了结核性脑炎患者。在加州脑炎报表中,结核病只占登记病例的不到1%[7]。这些差异与当地结核病流行病学有关。

9.3 病理生理学

大脑通过菌血症定植,原发感染位于呼吸道,有或者没有症状。少量结核杆菌进入血液,扩散到全身。大脑是可能发生转移的器官之一。在大脑中,结核分枝杆菌的作用与肺部相似[8-10]。

1. 3种细胞类型对于预防结核分枝杆菌是必不可少的:

(1) 巨噬细胞:吞噬细菌。结核分枝杆菌被巨噬细胞吞噬时,位于吞噬小体内。然后,它的脲酶停止酸化,从而阻止细菌在细胞内被消化。在吞噬小体中,抗原被提呈给Ⅱ类主要组织相容性复合体,刺激 $CD4^+$ T 细胞。由于抗原不会扩散到细胞质,所以它们不呈现在Ⅰ类主要组织相容性复合体中,顺便说一句,它们也不会刺激 $CD8^+$ T 细胞。

(2) $CD4^+$ T 淋巴细胞:分泌细胞因子 TH1(IFN-α)。

(3) $CD8^+$ T 淋巴细胞:分泌 IFN-α,能够溶解感染的巨噬细胞。

2. 肉芽肿是由以下物质制成的:

(1) 在其中心,巨噬细胞导致多核巨细胞增生。

(2) 在外周,T 和 B 淋巴细胞聚集。

坏死可发生在中心，导致干酪性脓肿，可钙化或液化。

初次感染和神经表现之间的延迟时间从几周（急性感染）到几年（复发）不等。

9.4 解剖病理学

脑膜渗出的特点是：最常见的部位是在脑底，最重要的是脑神经起源侵犯脉络丛，可扩散至脑室，脑叶炎症坏死可能与过敏反应有关。

血管病变与脑膜病变的程度相关，可能导致纤维蛋白坏死和血栓形成。

9.5 临床表现

脑炎的定义是根据文献中上述国际定义[1]。

通常情况下，结核性脑膜炎患者会出现一些特定的症状或情况。诊断上必须考虑延迟效应，与其他感染性脑炎相比，最常见的原因是多病例最初出现的神经症状较轻。在法国治疗的脑炎患者的一项研究报告中[3]，结核病患者出现全身症状和神经症状之间的中位延迟时间明显长于其他脑炎患者（10 天 vs. 2；$P<10^{-10}$）。在这项研究中，只有 20% 的患者有既往肺结核病史。11 名患者（55%）住在 ICU，其中 10 名接受机械通气，没有一例与持续的肺结核病有关。

9.6 生物学特征

结核病患者脑脊液中的蛋白水平高于其他病因[3]。结核组脑脊液蛋白中位数（2.1 g/L）明显高于其他脑炎组（0.8 g/L，$P=0.002$）。中位数为 150 个/mm³（范围 4~640 个/mm³）。16/18（89%）患者的血糖/血糖比值较低。

报告的诊断试验敏感性数据是从已发表的关于结核性脑膜炎的数据推断出来的，因为很少有关于结核性脑膜炎的研究[11]。

2004 年在越南对 132 例成人结核性脑膜炎患者进行了前瞻性研究。作者获得了 82% 的患者的微生物学诊断。镜检和脑脊液培养阳性率分别为 58% 和 71%[12]。在这项研究中，脑脊液镜检灵敏度的驱动因素是：① 每个患者的样本数量（尽管开始治疗，分析 1~3 个脑脊液样本的灵敏度在

37%～87%);② 可用的脑脊液体积(最多10～15 ml);③ 以及脑脊液沉淀物的检查。在一项涉及14个国家[13]的大型欧洲回顾性研究中,选择了506名确诊为中枢神经系统结核[镜检阳性和(或)特定培养基脑脊液培养阳性和(或)PCR阳性]的患者。作者观察到脑脊液细胞学结果为(320 ± 492)NC/mm³,以淋巴细胞为主($67\pm26\%$),脑脊液蛋白水平为(3.1 ± 4.2)g/L,脑脊液葡萄糖/血糖比值为0.28 ± 0.15。Lowenstein培养基培养灵敏度为72.6%,镜检灵敏度为27.3%。这可能是由于脑脊液中结核分枝杆菌接种量低,细菌定位于组织细胞而不是液体所致。

几位作者建议用脑脊液腺苷脱氨酶(adenosine deaminase, ADA)滴定作为鉴别结核性脑膜炎与其他细菌性脑膜炎的标准,但这项试验的效果尚有争议。荟萃分析作者报道ADA滴定诊断中枢神经系统结核的敏感性和特异性分别为79%和91%,阳性和阴性似然比分别为6.85和0.29[14]。另一项研究[15]报告了ADA滴定的灵敏度较低(55%)。然而,最近的欧洲研究报告,在常规治疗中只有41/137例(29.9%)ADA呈阳性[13]。到目前为止,最近的指南[16]不推荐这种测试。

PCR可作为诊断中枢神经系统结核分枝杆菌感染的较好工具。不幸的是,到目前为止,还没有针对脑脊液的标准化PCR,这项测试的性能与微生物实验室的经验和市场上使用的PCR有关。2013年,一项针对235 000名南非结核分枝杆菌脑膜炎患者的研究的作者观察到,定量Xpert MTB/RIF PCR与培养和(或)Amplicor PCR相比,与临床评分或脑脊液显微镜检查(革兰染色和金胺染色)相比,敏感性更高:分别为62%、30%和12%($P=0.001$)。以前对脑脊液样本进行离心的敏感性更好(82% vs. 47%),这需要3 ml的脑脊液(而不是1 ml)。南非是结核病流行国家,Xpert MTB/RIF试验的PPV和NPV分别为90%和77%。2014年发表的一项对8项研究的荟萃分析显示,与培养相比,脑脊液中Xpert MTB/RIF检测的敏感性和特异性分别为81%和98%[18]。这项多中心欧洲研究的作者观察到结核分枝杆菌PCR的敏感度为57.3%[15]。通过对异种PCR技术(Cobas®Amplicor, Grenzach-Wyhlen,德国罗氏)、RT-PCR(ProbeTec®,Becton Dickinson,英国牛津)、GeneProof®(GeneProof, Brno,捷克共和国)和GeneXpert®(Cepheid,桑尼维尔,美国加利福尼亚州)的分析来测量灵敏度,不同方法的应用使得无法评估这些技术的灵敏度。欧洲作者还强调了进行血液IGRA测试(Quantiferon®-TB金试管测试)的可能性,并报告了良好的结果:41

项测试中有 37 项阳性结果(敏感度为 90.2%)。

9.7 影像学

脑 MRI 是诊断脑炎的最好工具,只有在 MRI 不能检查的情况下才应该使用 CT 扫描[16]。

除了脑脓肿或肉芽肿性病变外,结核性脑炎没有特殊的影像。在最近的研究[3]中,17 名患者中有 8 名入院时 CT 扫描和 MRI 检查正常,这意味着在图像正常的情况下不可能排除结核病的诊断。

9.8 治疗

9.8.1 标准

延迟结核性脑炎患者的抗菌治疗与增加病死率和神经后遗症的风险相关[19]。最常见的经验性治疗的原因是因为难以确定最终诊断(基于细菌学或组织学数据)和快速诊断试验的低灵敏度[20]。在确诊前,临床恶化或迅速好转不应导致早期停药。人们应该记住,特定的抗结核治疗可能与长时间起作用有关,特别是在出现严重脑损伤的患者中。因此,除非最终的准确诊断被确定,否则经验性治疗应该在标准治疗期内持续实施[21]。一些人建议进行为期 6 个月的强化治疗[22]。然而,标准的推荐治疗方法是通常的 4 种药物(利福平、异烟肼、吡嗪酰胺和乙胺丁醇)联合治疗 2 个月,然后进行双重联合治疗,总疗程为 9~12 个月[23-25]。意外中断治疗是结核性脑炎患者病死率的独立危险因素[26],临床研究支持标准的长期治疗。

异烟肼是一种快速杀菌剂,具有良好的脑脊液扩散[27]。通常剂量[3~5 mg/(kg·d)]给药后,脑脊液中异烟肼的浓度是结核分枝杆菌最低抑菌浓度的 10~15 倍[28]。几位作者建议将异烟肼的剂量增加到 5 mg/(kg·d)以上,即儿童 10~20 mg/(kg·d)。然而,其出色的脑脊液扩散并不支持在结核分枝杆菌敏感株的情况下增加剂量。因此,异烟肼可以通过快速静脉给药,辅以吡哆醇补充(1 次 1 剂)。

利福平没有达到如此重要的脑脊液水平:它们低于血清浓度的 30%[27]。然而,与对利福平耐药的结核性脑炎相关的病死率证实了这种抗生素是治疗的关键合作伙伴[29]。考虑到利福平的中枢神经系统弥散性较低,儿童服用利福平的剂量为 20 mg/(kg·d),耐受性良好。类似的剂量也用于骨和关节感染,没有任何安全问题。在患有结核性脑炎的患者中,除了使用异烟肼、吡嗪酰胺和皮质激素的标准治疗外,使用更高剂量的利福平(600 mg 静脉注射 vs. 450 mg/口服)和莫西沙星(800 mg vs. 400 mg/口服)对改善病死率没有好处[30]。综合以上数据,推荐常规剂量利福平[10 mg/(kg·d)]。

吡嗪酰胺具有良好的口服生物利用度和良好的脑脊液分布[31]。儿童 40 mg/(kg·d),成人 30 mg/(kg·d),不超过 1.5 g/d[22]。

乙胺丁醇通常被建议放在第四位[27],尽管它在中枢神经系统的扩散很差(特别是在没有炎症的情况下)。

9.8.2 抗结核分枝杆菌

氟喹诺酮类药物是一种选择,特别是在处理对"通常"4 种药物组合中包括的一种分子的耐药性或禁忌证时。然而,孕妇或哺乳期妇女以及儿童的长期治疗都必须避免[32]。在氟喹诺酮类药物中,莫西沙星被认为具有最好的活性[33-35]。对异烟肼单一耐药(高度耐药),建议用氟喹诺酮替代异烟肼,疗程 2 个月,然后继续与利福平、吡嗪酰胺、氟喹诺酮三联用药,总疗程 12 个月。对于对异烟肼的低水平耐药性,仍应继续开药方。对于利福平的单一耐药,建议用氟喹诺酮替代利福平,疗程 2 个月,然后继续与异烟肼、吡嗪酰胺和氟喹诺酮三联用药,总疗程为 18 个月[23]。利奈唑胺也已被成功使用[36],但当与二线治疗相结合时,它仅限于多重耐药菌株的病例。

9.8.3 辅助治疗

皮质激素可以改善与非感染性疾病(脑水肿、血管炎)相关的预后。增加皮质激素治疗是基于对结核性脑膜炎的研究结果的推断,这些研究表明,非 HIV 感染患者必须接受皮质激素和抗结核治疗,而不考虑疾病的严重程度[26,37],这一点是基于对结核性脑膜炎的研究结果的推断,这些研究表明,非 HIV 感染患者必须接受带有抗结核治疗的皮质激素治疗,而不考虑疾病的严重程度[26,37]。通常推荐的地塞米松或泼尼松剂量成人为 0.4 mg/(kg·d),儿童为 0.6 mg/(kg·d)。糖皮质激素治疗通常持续 4 周,然后在 4 周以上逐步脱机。英国指南建议在观察到神经体征时使用地塞米松 0.4 mg/(kg·d)，在没有意识障碍或局灶性神经体征的情况下使用 0.3 mg/(kg·d)[23]。

在使用糖皮质激素或免疫重建炎症综合征的持续性脑水肿的情况下，一些报告了使用干扰素-γ[38]、英夫利昔单抗（抗 TNF）[39]和沙利度胺[40]的临床病例研究。阿司匹林可以对分枝杆菌感染有抗炎作用（抑制二十烷类化合物和促炎 TNF 的表达）[41]。最近两项研究的作者表明，阿司匹林降低了表现为结核性脑膜炎（特别是 LTA4H 基因型）的患者偏瘫、中风和病死的发生率[42,43]。

9.8.4 手术

对于结核性脑炎，脑积水和脑脓肿是紧急神经外科手术的主要适应证。它的目的是在脑脓肿的情况下降低颅内压和接种细菌[44]。外科引流也可能是一种诊断工具（组织学、培养和结核分枝杆菌药敏试验）。当怀疑有生命危险的脑积水时，应紧急进行脑室外引流。

9.9 结果和预后

在法国的研究[3]中，他们没有包括感染多重耐药菌株的患者。然而，有 6 名患者（33%）在住院期间死亡。出院时有 10 例（78.6%）有持续性神经症状。尽管没有多重耐药的结核分枝杆菌菌株，但与其他病因相比，在本系列中，结核性脑炎患者的病死率很高。其他病因（包括单纯疱疹病毒）的病死率为 9%，差异有统计学意义。

一项多中心多国研究的作者[45]提出了结核性脑膜炎不良结局的评分标准。33%的患者报告了不良的结果，与脑炎的观察结果严格相似，也就是说，这两个发现都得到了相当大的验证。他们使用以下项目来提供严重程度指数，与结果呈线性相关：意识改变、意识改变加上恶心、呕吐、糖尿病、免疫抑制、神经功能障碍、脑积水和血管炎。这一评分在脑炎中没有得到验证，但它很可能是到目前为止，评估预后的一个基础。

尽管在一个高收入国家进行管理，结核性脑炎往往预后不佳，即使是在敏感菌株的情况下也是如此。

9.10 结论

在高收入国家,结核性脑炎仍然是一种负担。这是一种常见的病因,哪怕接受了规范的治疗,很难评估低收入患者的疗效。

参考文献

[1] Venkatesan A, Tunkel AR, Bloch KC, Lauring AS, Sejvar J, Bitnun A, Stahl J-P, Mailles A, Drebot M, Rupprecht CE, Yoder J, Cope JR, Wilson MR, Whitley RJ, Sullivan J, Granerod J, Jones C, Eastwood K, Ward KN, Durrheim DN, Solbrig MV, Guo-Dong L, Glaser CA. Case definitions, diagnostic algorithms, and priorities in encephalitis: consensus statement of the international encephalitis consortium. Clin Infect Dis. 2013; 57(8): 1114-1128.

[2] Sotgiu G, Falzon D, Hollo V, KoÈdmoÈn C, Lefebvre N, Dadu A, van der Werf M. Determinants of site of tuberculosis disease: An analysis of European surveillance data from 2003 to 2014. Plos One. 2017; https://doi.org/10.1371/journal.pone.0186499.

[3] Honnorat E, De Broucker T, Mailles A, Stahl JP. Encephalitis due to Mycobacterium tuberculosis in France. Med Mal Infect. 2013; 43(6): 230-238.

[4] Cobo F, Salas-Coronas J, Cabezas-Fernandez MT, Vazquez-Villegas J, Cabeza-Barrera MI, Soriano-Perez MJ. Infectious diseases in immigrant population related to the time of residence in Spain. J Immigr Minor Health. 2016; 18: 8-15.

[5] Mailles A, Stahl J-P. Infectious encephalitis in France in 2007: a national prospective study. Clin Infect Dis. 2009; 49: 1838-1847.

[6] Granerod J, Ambrose HE, Davies NWS, Clewley JP, Walsh AL, Morgan D, et al. Causes of encephalitis and 5 differences in their clinical presentations in England: a multicentre, population-based prospective study. Lancet Infect Dis. 2010; 10(12): 835-844.

[7] Christie LJ, Loeffler AM, Honarmand S, Flood JM, Baxter R, Jacobson S, Alexander R, Glaser CA. Diagnostic challenges of central nervous system tuberculosis. Emerg Infect Dis. 2008; 14(9): 1473-1475.

[8] Algood HM, Lin PL, Flynn JL. Tumor necrosis factor and chemokine interactions in the formation and maintenance of granulomas in tuberculosis. Clin Infect Dis. 2005; 41(Suppl 3): S189-193.

[9] Edwards D, et al. The immunology of mycobacterial diseases. Am Rev Respir Dis. 1986; 134: 1062-1071.

[10] Friedland JS. Cytokines, phagocytosis, and mycobacterium tuberculosis. *Lymphokine Cytokine Res*. 1993; 12: 127-133.

[11] Fillatre P, Crabol Y, Morand P, Piroth L, Honnorat J, Stahl JP, Lecuit M. Infectious encephalitis: Management without etiological diagnosis 48 hours after

onset. Med Mal Infect. 2017; 47: 236-251.
[12] Thwaites GE, Chau TTH, Farrar JJ. Improving the bacteriological diagnosis of tuberculous meningitis. J Clin Microbiol. 2004; 42(1): 378-379.
[13] Erdem H, Ozturk Engin D, Elaldi N, Gulsun S, Sengoz G, Crisan A, et al. The microbiological diagnosis of tuberculous meningitis: results of Haydarpasal study. Clin Microbiol Infect. 2014; 20(10): O600-608.
[14] Xu HB, Jiang RH, Li L, Sha W, Xiao HP. Diagnostic value of adenosine deaminase in cerebrospinal fluid for tuberculous meningitis: a meta-analysis. Int J Tuberc Lung Dis. 2010; 14(11): 1382-1387.
[15] Solari L, Soto A, Agapito JC, Acurio V, Vargas D, Battaglioli T, et al. The validity of cerebrospinal fluid parameters for the diagnosis of tuberculous meningitis. Int J Infect Dis. 2013; 17(12): e1111-1115.
[16] Stahl JP, Azouvi P, Bruneel F, De Broucker T, Duval X, Fantin B, Girard N, Herrmann JL, Honnorat J, et al. Guidelines on the management of infectious encephalitis in adults. Med Mal Infect. 2017; 47(3): 179-194.
[17] Patel VB, Theron G, Lenders L, Matinyena B, Connolly C, Singh R, et al. Diagnostic accuracy of quantitative PCR (Xpert MTB/RIF) for tuberculous meningitis in a high burden setting: a prospective study. PLoS Med. 2013; 10 (10): e1001536.
[18] Denkinger CM, Schumacher SG, Boehme CC, Dendukuri N, Pai M, Steingart KR. Xpert MTB/RIF assay for the diagnosis of extrapulmonary tuberculosis: a systematic review and meta-analysis. Eur Respir J. 2014; 44(2): 435-446.
[19] Goulenok T, Buzelé R, Duval X, Bruneel F, Stahl JP, Fantin B. Management of adult infectious encephalitis in metropolitan France. Med Mal Infect. 2017; 47: 206-220.
[20] Chiang SS, Khan FA, Milstein MB, Tolman AW, Benedetti A, Starke JR, et al. Treatment outcomes of childhood tuberculous meningitis: a systematic review and meta-analysis. Lancet Infect Dis. 2014; 14(10): 947-957.
[21] Thwaites GE, van Toorn R, Schoeman J. Tuberculous meningitis: more questions, still too few answers. Lancet Neurol. 2013; 12(10): 999-1010.
[22] Donald PR, Schoeman JF, Van Zyl LE, De Villiers JN, Pretorius M, Springer P. Intensive short course chemotherapy in the management of tuberculous meningitis. Int J Tuberc Lung Dis. 1998; 2(9): 704-711.
[23] Thwaites G, Fisher M, Hemingway C, Scott G, Solomon T, Innes J. British Infection Society guidelines for the diagnosis and treatment of tuberculosis of the central nervous system in adults and children. J Infect. 2009; 59(3): 167-187.
[24] American Thoracic Society, Center for Disease Control and Prevention, Infectious Disease Society of America. Treatment of tuberculosis. MMWR Morb Mortal Wkly Rep. 2003; 52(RR-11): 1-77.
[25] Heemskerk AD, Bang ND, Mai NT, Chau TT, Phu NH, Loc PP, et al. Intensified antituberculosis therapy in adults with tuberculous meningitis. N Engl J Med. 2016; 374(2): 124-134.
[26] Thwaites GE, Nguyen DB, Nguyen HD, Hoang TQ, Do TT, Nguyen TC, et al. Dexamethasone for the treatment of tuberculous meningitis in adolescents and

adults. N Engl J Med. 2004; 351(17): 1741-1751.
[27] Ellard GA, Humphries MJ, Allen BW. Cerebrospinal fluid drug concentrations and the treatment of tuberculous meningitis. Am Rev Respir Dis. 1993; 148(3): 650-655.
[28] Kaojarern S, Supmonchai K, Phuapradit P, Mokkhavesa C. Clin Pharmacol Ther. 1991; 49(1): 6-12.
[29] Thwaites GE, Lan NT, Dung NH, Quy HT, Oanh DT, Thoa NT, et al. Effect of antituberculosis drug resistance on response to treatment and outcome in adults with tuberculous meningitis. J Infect Dis. 2005; 192(1): 79-88.
[30] Ruslami R, Ganiem AR, Dian S, Apriani L, Achmad TH, van der Ven AJ, et al. Intensified regimen containing rifampicin and moxifloxacin for tuberculous meningitis: an open-label, randomised controlled phase 2 trial. Lancet Infect Dis. 2013; 13(1): 27-35.
[31] Ellard GA, Humphries MJ, Gabriel M, Teoh R. Penetration of pyrazinamide into the cerebrospinal fluid in tuberculous meningitis. Br Med J (Clin Res Ed). 1987; 294(6567): 284-285.
[32] Mehlhorn AJ, Brown DA. Safety concerns with fluoroquinolones. Ann Pharmacother. 2007; 41(11): 1859-1866.
[33] Thwaites GE, Bhavnani SM, Chau TT, Hammel JP, Torok ME, Van Wart SA, et al. Randomized pharmacokinetic and pharmacodynamic comparison of fluoroquinolones for tuberculous meningitis. Antimicrob Agents Chemother. 2011; 55(7): 3244-3253.
[34] Alffenaar JW, van Altena R, Bokkerink HJ, Luijckx GJ, van Soolingen D, Aarnoutse RE, et al. Pharmacokinetics of moxifloxacin in cerebrospinal fluid and plasma in patients with tuberculous meningitis. Clin Infect Dis. 2009; 49(7): 1080-1082.
[35] Heemskerk AD. Intensified treatment with high-dose Rifampicin and Levofloxacin compared to standard treatment for adult patients with Tuberculous Meningitis (TBM-IT): protocol for a randomized controlled trial. Trials. 2011; 12: 25.
[36] Yu HY, Hu FS, Xiang DR, Sheng JF. Clinical management of tuberculous meningitis: experiences of 42 cases and literature review. Neurol Sci. 2014; 35(2): 303-305.
[37] Prasad K, Singh MB. Corticosteroids for managing tuberculous meningitis. Cochrane Database Syst Rev. 2008; (1): CD002244.
[38] Coulter JB, Baretto RL, Mallucci CL, Romano MI, Abernethy LJ, Isherwood DM, et al. Tuberculous meningitis: protracted course and clinical response to interferon gamma. Lancet Infect Dis. 2007; 7(3): 225-232.
[39] Blackmore TK, Manning L, Taylor WJ, Wallis RS. Therapeutic use of infliximab in tuberculosis to control severe paradoxical reaction of the brain and lymph nodes. Clin Infect Dis. 2008; 47(10): e83-85.
[40] Roberts MT, Mendelson M, Meyer P, Carmichael A, Lever AM. The use of thalidomide in the treatment of intracranial tuberculomas in adults: two case reports. J Infect. 2003; 47(3): 251-255.
[41] Tobin DM, Roca FJ, Oh SF, McFarland R, Vickery TW, Ray JP, et al. Host genotype-specific therapies can optimize the inflammatory response to mycobacterial

infections. Cell. 2012; 148(3): 434-446.
[42] Misra UK, Kalita J, Nair PP. Role of aspirin in tuberculous meningitis: a randomized open-label placebo-controlled trial. J Neurol Sci. 2010; 293(1-2): 12-17.
[43] Schoeman JF, Janse van Rensburg A, Laubscher JA, Springer P. The role of aspirin in childhood tuberculous meningitis. J Child Neurol. 2011; 26(8): 956-962.
[44] Cardenas G, Soto-Hernandez JL, Orozco RV, Silva EG, Revuelta R, Amador JL. Tuberculous brain abscesses in immunocompetent patients: management and outcome. Neurosurgery. 2010; 67(4): 1081-1087.
[45] Erdem H, Ozturk-Engin D, Tireli H, Kilicoglu G, Defres S, Gulsun S, Sengoz G, Crisan A, Johansen IS, et al. Hamsi scoring in the prediction of unfavorable outcomes from tuberculous meningitis: results of Haydarpasa-II study. J Neurol. 2015; 262(4): 890-898.

10
脊柱结核

盖达·艾哈迈德·谢哈塔

10.1 前言

脊柱感染包括主要影响：① 脊髓；② 神经根和脑膜；③ 椎骨、椎间盘和硬膜外间隙的感染。它们大致分为化脓性和非化脓性，前者包括椎体骨髓炎和椎间盘炎，后者包括寄生性、真菌性和结节性感染。

10.2 定义

结核病是影响人类的最古老的病理疾病之一。它可以影响肺部以外的几个组织。5%的结核病例影响骨骼系统，其中50%位于脊柱[1]，并引起一种椎间关节结核性关节炎。脊柱结核（spinal tuberculosis，STB）也被称为波特病，以珀西瓦尔·波特的名字命名，他在1779年发表了对它的第一个描述[2]。

10.3 流行病学

结核病是一个全球性的健康问题，影响着世界1/3的人口[3]。它是一种广泛的疾病，每年有870万新病例，世界范围内的结核病发病率与HIV发病率同步上升[4]。不仅在非洲和亚洲，而且在欧洲国家都见证了结核病的增加。此外，结核病在感染性死亡原因中排名第二，仅次于HIV感染。因此，结核病仍然是全世界发病率和病死率的重要原因[5]。据报告，土耳其是结核病低发病率国家[3]。

当考虑到EPTB尤其是STB流行病学时，10%～35%的EPTB病例考虑STB[6]。2016年，据估计，STB约占所有结核病病例的2%，约占EPTB

病例的 15%[7]。

10.4 进展中的脊柱结核的危险因素

STB 的易感因素很多,包括既往的结核病感染和营养不良[8]。STB 风险增加的人群包括免疫受损人群(患有 HIV、淋巴瘤、白血病或器官移植)、糖尿病患者、儿童、老年人、酗酒者、社会经济地位低下者、治疗依从性差的人、来自发展中国家的移民、囚犯、疗养院居民、医护人员和无家可归者[9,10]。此外,皮肤、泌尿生殖道、胃肠道或呼吸道感染灶的血液学播种被认为是 STB 的重要危险因素[11]。

10.5 病理生理学

STB 有两种类型:经典型(或脊柱椎间盘炎)和一种日益常见的非典型类型,即无椎间盘受累的脊柱炎[12]。在成人中,椎间盘的受累是从邻近的感染椎体扩散的次要原因,而在儿童中,主要是由于椎间盘的血管化性质所致。在成人中,椎间盘的受累是次要的,而在儿童中,这主要是由于椎间盘的血管化性质造成的。

脊柱结核的基本病变是骨髓炎和关节炎的组合,通常累及不止一个椎骨。靠近软骨板的椎体前方通常受累[13]。STB 可包括以下任何一种:进行性骨质破坏,导致脊椎塌陷和后凸,脓肿导致椎管狭窄,冷脓肿形成(由于感染延伸到邻近韧带和软组织),或肉芽组织或直接侵犯硬脑膜,导致脊髓受压。这些事件会导致不同的神经缺陷[8,12,13]。

10.6 诊断

诊断依据是病史、脊柱影像学检查、胸部 X 线片、胸部 CT 扫描和实验室检查,如白细胞计数和纯化蛋白衍生物试验。

临床特点

临床病程

脊柱受累是结核分枝杆菌向椎体松质骨组织血源性扩散的结果[7]。主要感染部位来自肺部病灶或另一肺外病灶,如胃肠道或淋巴结[8]。

临床表现

STB 的诊断延误是很常见的[7]。STB 患者可能会出现各种各样的症状[14]。从发病到确诊的平均时间为 1 年零 7 个月。通常情况下,症状的出现是隐匿的,疾病进展缓慢。诊断前症状的持续时间可能从 2 周到几年不等[15]。

关于 STB 患者的性别差异,53% 的 STB 患者是男性[7]。临床表现和体检结果取决于疾病的部位和阶段、并发症的存在和体质症状[16]。最常见的症状是局灶性背痛、发烧、体重减轻和神经异常,如肠、膀胱功能障碍的运动或感觉根影响,以及截瘫[7]。

此外,患者有活动性结核病的全身症状,包括咳嗽、呼吸急促、发烧、发冷和盗汗。

脊柱结核术后并发症分析

神经缺陷的发生率为 23%~76%[7]。

并发症包括脊髓空洞症、永久性神经缺陷和脊柱骨缺损[17]。截瘫被认为是 STB 最具破坏性的并发症。

实验室检查

STB 需要进行血液学检查,如全血细胞计数、血细胞沉降率、酶联免疫吸附试验和聚合酶链反应(PCR)[7]。

微生物学证据至少包括以下一项:在血液、骨、骨髓、深层软组织和(或)(椎旁、硬膜外或腰大肌)脓肿标本中分离出结核分枝杆菌;从骨、骨髓、深层软组织和(或)(椎旁、硬膜外或腰大肌)脓肿或任何无菌身体组织中分离出抗酸杆菌。抗酸杆菌染色的骨组织或脓肿样本,培养分离出的分枝杆菌,以及 CT 引导或超声引导的穿刺活检或手术活检也被广泛使用[7,15,18]。这可以通过使用 Ziehl-Neelsen 染色来完成。另外,采用 Ziehl-Neelsen 染色快速培养,PCR 检测结核分枝杆菌复合体[3,7,19]。

一种基于生物标志物的非组织快速检测方法

用两种分枝杆菌蛋白-培养滤液蛋白-10 和早期分泌型抗原靶标-6 对

结核免疫学诊断工具的准确性进行了评估[20]。以 CFP10/ESAT6 融合蛋白为抗原的酶联免疫斑点试验(enzyme-linked immunospot，ELISPOT)具有较高的敏感性和特异性，是 STB 辅助诊断的有效方法[20]。这些免疫诊断试验，全血干扰素-g(IFN-g)酶联免疫吸附试验 Quantiferon-TB Gold (Cellestis Ltd.，Chadstone，VIC，澳大利亚)和酶联免疫斑点试验 T-SPOT.TB(牛津免疫技术公司,牛津,英国)，可以定量测量结核分枝杆菌特异性免疫优势抗原特异性淋巴细胞产生 IFN-g 的数量,这些淋巴细胞是由病原体的 Rd1 区域编码的。另一种商品化的 IFN-g 释放试验(IGRA)，Quantiferon-TB Gold in-tube test(QFTGIT)(Cellestis Ltd.)，能够测定针对结核免疫优势抗原早期分泌物抗原靶标-6 和培养滤液蛋白-10 的特异性 IFN-g 的产生[7]。

影像学诊断

脊柱结核通常表现为结核性脑膜炎(tuberculous meningitis，TBM)，很少表现为髓内结核球[9]。然而,平片最初是在怀疑患有 STB 的患者中进行的,平片图像显示了动脉瘤现象的鸟巢外观特征[21]。

磁共振成像

磁共振成像(MRI)异常包括起源于椎体终板的脊柱病变,累及椎体前角,显示椎体下扩散的证据,显示多个椎体但保留椎间盘,显示广泛的椎旁脓肿形成,脓肿钙化,以及椎体破坏或椎体塌陷[9,21]。

此外,还有广泛的椎旁脓肿形成和脓肿钙化[9]。CT 在确定软组织脓肿的形状和钙化方面比平片更有效,因为 CT 能更好地显示不规则溶解性病变、硬化、椎间盘塌陷和骨周破坏的骨质细节。

要使放射透明病变在平片图像上可见,必须有 30% 的骨矿物质丢失[15]。

正电子发射断层扫描(PET)可用于鉴别 STB 和其他化脓性脊柱炎[22]。MRI 可早期发现 STB,可减少 STB 并发症。只有在活检或培养结果的基础上才能做出确认性诊断[9]。

10.7 脊柱结核的分类

库马尔(Kumar)介绍了基于受累部位和疾病分期的后部 STB 的 4 点分类[23]。归因于这种分类系统的一个最重要的限制是它只包括后部 STB，这是相对罕见的。

梅塔（Mehta）和博赫拉吉（Bhojraj）引入了一种新的STB分类系统，使用MRI结果进行分类。他们根据所采用的手术技术将患者分成4组。A组：前路病变稳定，无后凸畸形；B组包括全局病变、后凸畸形和不稳定的患者；C组患者由于内科并发症和可能的麻醉并发症，前部或全局性病变，以及经胸手术的手术风险很高；最后，D组患者仅需后路减压即可获得孤立的后路病变[23,24]。这种分类只对胸部病变进行分类，这是该系统最重要的限制[13]。

10.8 治疗

抗结核药物在STB患者的康复和应答中起主要作用[25]。在没有神经功能障碍、不稳定和畸形的情况下，无论是否存在椎旁脓肿，这些药物的疗效已经在几项关于STB治疗的研究中得到证明[26]。充分和早期的药物治疗可以预防严重的并发症[27]。利福平、异烟肼、乙胺丁醇和吡嗪酰胺联合治疗2个月，然后利福平和异烟肼联合治疗6个月、9个月、12个月或18个月，是治疗STB最常用的方案[17,26,27]。短程化疗方案已经被证明有很好的效果，除了在15岁以下的患者和那些初始后凸角度超过30度且后凸显著增加的患者[28]。单独接受医疗治疗的患者可以接受CT引导下的靶区引流[7]。

耐多药结核病被定义为对利福平和异烟肼耐药的生物体[25]。如果临床或放射学没有改善，出现新的病变或冷脓肿，或尽管接受了3~5个月的治疗，骨质破坏增加，就会检测到这种耐药性[25]。耐多药结核病是一个全球性的问题；在所有新病例中有3%遇到这种情况，在再治疗病例中有12%遇到这种情况[13]。耐多药结核病的推荐治疗至少24个月，平均使用6种抗结核药物[29]。WHO最新的指南建议使用5种预计在最初强化阶段有效的药物，以及4种可能在持续阶段有效的药物。初期疗程为6~9个月，总疗程为20~24个月[29]。密切监测患者不良反应的发展是必要的[25,29]。

10.8.1 手术治疗

就诊时的神经状态是决定治疗决策和患者预后的关键因素。如果影像学结果提示存在STB,手术治疗的决定应基于对治疗失败风险的评估,以及根据脊柱炎分级系统[30]。通常需要手术来减压[31]、矫正脊柱后凸和维持脊柱稳定性[31,32]。关于理想的手术入路还存在争议。前入路可以直接进入感染部位,这对清创很有帮助。然而,在脊柱后凸矫正和维持脊柱稳定性方面,单一前路手术可能导致不满意的结果[33]。单一后路手术在脊柱后凸矫正和维持脊柱稳定性方面显示出优势,但它不能完全清除椎体前方的感染病变[32]。因此,前路清创/植骨和后路内固定相结合,克服了单纯通过前路或后路手术的缺点,已成为治疗STB的常见选择[32]。随着脊柱微创外科的发展,后路经皮内固定技术也被用于丰富前路清创/植骨/后路内固定的手术方法[32]。

10.8.2 预后

耐多药结核病治疗成功或失败的决定因素是:① 化疗后6个月的临床逐步改善;② 治疗期间放射学的改善;③ 结核分枝杆菌菌株对最多3种抗结核药物和最多4种二线药物的抗药性;④ 治疗期间药物方案不变[29]。

手术干预前需要明确一些预后因素。脊柱后凸可以定义为负Cobb角的发生,在骨质破坏的基础上可以出现在腰椎水平。就生理脊柱曲线而言,腰椎保持前凸曲线,Cobb角范围为30°～50°。137例STB引起的脊柱后凸,因骨质破坏,腰椎STB预后的前凸曲线变为后凸,Cobb角变为负值[30]。姚等人[34]确定非瘫痪、症状持续时间较短、椎体受累较少和经皮内固定是术后恢复的有利预后因素。术后早期(1～3个月),经皮内固定组[日本骨科协会(JOA)]评分高于开放内固定组,但远期(6～24个月)JOA评分无明显差异。此外,经皮内固定治疗的患者手术时间较短。

参考文献

[1] Graves VB, Schreiber MH. Tuberculous psoas muscle abscess. J Can Assoc Radiol. 1973; 24(3): 268-271.
[2] Benli IT, Kis M, Akalin S, Citak M, Kanevetci S, Duman E. The results of anterior radical debridement and anterior instrumentation in Pott's disease and comparison with other surgical techniques. Kobe J Med Sci. 2000; 46(1-2): 39-68.
[3] Batirel A, Erdem H, Sengoz G, Pehlivanoglu F, Ramosaco E, Gulsun S, et al. The course of spinal tuberculosis (Pott disease): results of the multinational,

multicentre Backbone-2 study. Clin Microbiol Infect. 2015; 21(11): 1008 e9-e18.
[4] Cohen KA, Abeel T, Manson McGuire A, Desjardins CA, Munsamy V, Shea TP, et al. Evolution of extensively drug-resistant tuberculosis over four decades: whole genome sequencing and dating analysis of *Mycobacterium tuberculosis* isolates from KwaZulu-Natal. PLoS Med. 2015; 12(9): e1001880.
[5] Alrajhi AA, Al-Barrak AM. Extrapulmonary tuberculosis, epidemiology and patterns in Saudi Arabia. Saudi Med J. 2002; 23(5): 503-508.
[6] Peto HM, Pratt RH, Harrington TA, Lobue PA, Armstrong LR. Epidemiology of extrapulmonary tuberculosis in the United States, 1993-2006. Clin Infect Dis. 2009; 49(9): 1350-1357.
[7] Chen CH, Chen YM, Lee CW, Chang YJ, Cheng CY, Hung JK. Early diagnosis of spinal tuberculosis. J Formos Med Assoc. 2016; 115(10): 825-836.
[8] Boachie-Adjei O, Squillante RG. Tuberculosis of the spine. Orthop Clin North Am. 1996; 27(1): 95-103.
[9] Gambhir S, Ravina M, Rangan K, Dixit M, Barai S, Bomanji J, et al. Imaging in extrapulmonary tuberculosis. Int J Infect Dis. 2017; 56: 237-247.
[10] Maclean KA, Becker AK, Chang SD, Harris AC. Extrapulmonary tuberculosis: imaging features beyond the chest. Can Assoc Radiol J. 2013; 64(4): 319-324.
[11] Tyagi R. Spinal infections in children: a review. J Orthop. 2016; 13(4): 254-258.
[12] Pertuiset E, Beaudreuil L, Liote F, editors. Spinal tuberculosis in adults. A study of 103 cases in a developed. country, 1980-1994. Medicine (Baltimore) 1999; 78 (5): 309-320.
[13] Rasouli MR, Mirkoohi M, Vaccaro AR, Yarandi KK, Rahimi-Movaghar V. Spinal tuberculosis: diagnosis and management. Asian Spine J. 2012; 6(4): 294-308.
[14] Kaloostian PE, Gokaslan ZL. Current management of spinal tuberculosis: a multimodal approach. World Neurosurg. 2013; 80(1-2): 64-65.
[15] Ansari S, Amanullah MF, Ahmad K, Rauniyar RK. Pott's spine: diagnostic imaging modalities and technology advancements. N Am J Med Sci. 2013; 5(7): 404-411.
[16] Nussbaum ES, Rockswold GL, Bergman TA, Erickson DL, Seljeskog EL. Spinal tuberculosis: a diagnostic and management challenge. J Neurosurg. 1995; 83(2): 243-247.
[17] Chen YH, Lin C, Harnod T, Wu WT, Yu JC, Chen CH. Treatment modalities for tuberculosis of the spine: 22 years' experience in east Taiwan. Formos J Surg. 2013; 46: 189-194.
[18] Mok JH, Kim KU, Park HK, Lee MK. Extensively drug-resistant tuberculosis presenting as primary lymphadenitis eroding into the trachea in an immunocompetent patient. J Formos Med Assoc. 2014; 113(10): 764-765.
[19] Alli OA, Ogbolu OD, Alaka OO. Direct molecular detection of *Mycobacterium tuberculosis* complex from clinical samples — an adjunct to cultural method of laboratory diagnosis of tuberculosis. N Am J Med Sci. 2011; 3(6): 281-288.
[20] Yuan K, Liang D, Wu XQ, Yao ZS, Jin DX, Yang ZD, et al. Diagnostic value of enzyme-linked immunospot assay using CFP10/ESAT6 fusion protein as antigen in spinal tuberculosis. Zhongguo Yi Xue Ke Xue Yuan Xue Bao. 2015; 37(1): 44-49.

[21] Alvi AA, Raees A, Khan Rehmani MA, Aslam HM, Saleem S, Ashraf J. Magnetic resonance image findings of spinal tuberclosis at first presentation. Int Arch Med. 2014; 7(1): 12.

[22] Lee IS, Lee JS, Kim SJ, Jun S, Suh KT. Fluorine-18-fluorodeoxyglucose positron emission tomography/computed tomography imaging in pyogenic and tuberculous spondylitis: preliminary study. J Comput Assist Tomogr. 2009; 33 (4): 587-592.

[23] Kumar K. A clinical study and classification of posterior spinal tuberculosis. Int Orthop. 1985; 9(3): 147-152.

[24] Mehta JS, Bhojraj SY. Tuberculosis of the thoracic spine: a classification based on the selection of surgical strategies. J Bone Joint Surg. 2001; 83(6): 859-863.

[25] Jain AK. Tuberculosis of the spine: a fresh look at an old disease. J Bone Joint Surg. 2010; 92(7): 905-913.

[26] Kotil K, Alan MS, Bilge T. Medical management of Pott disease in the thoracic and lumbar spine: a prospective clinical study. J Neurosurg Spine. 2007; 6(3): 222-228.

[27] Alothman A, Memish ZA, Awada A, Al-Mahmood S, Al-Sadoon S, Rahman MM, et al. Tuberculous spondylitis: analysis of 69 cases from Saudi Arabia. Spine. 2001; 26(24): E565-570.

[28] Parthasarathy R, Sriram K, Santha T, Prabhakar R, Somasundaram PR, Sivasubramanian S. Short-course chemotherapy for tuberculosis of the spine. A comparison between ambulant treatment and radical surgery — ten-year report. J Bone Joint Surg. 1999; 81(3): 464-471.

[29] Pawar UM, Kundnani V, Agashe V, Nene A, Nene A. Multidrug-resistant tuberculosis of the spine — is it the beginning of the end? A study of twenty-five culture proven multidrug-resistant tuberculosis spine patients. Spine. 2009; 34 (22): E806-810.

[30] Turgut M. Spinal tuberculosis (Pott's disease): its clinical presentation, surgical management, and outcome. A survey study on 694 patients. Neurosurg Rev 2001; 24(1): 8-13. doi: 10.1007/PL00011973.

[31] Ma YZ, Cui X, Li HW, Chen X, Cai XJ, Bai YB. Outcomes of anterior and posterior instrumentation under different surgical procedures for treating thoracic and lumbar spinal tuberculosis in adults. Int Orthop. 2012; 36(2): 299-305.

[32] Wang X, Pang X, Wu P, Luo C, Shen X. One-stage anterior debridement, bone grafting and posterior instrumentation vs. single posterior debridement, bone grafting, and instrumentation for the treatment of thoracic and lumbar spinal tuberculosis. Eur Spine J. 2014; 23(4): 830-837.

[33] Benli IT, Kaya A, Acaroglu E. Anterior instrumentation in tuberculous spondylitis: is it effective and safe? Clin Orthop Relat Res. 2007; 460: 108-116.

[34] Yao Y, Zhang H, Liu H, Zhang Z, Tang Y, Zhou Y. Prognostic factors for recovery after anterior debridement/bone grafting and posterior instrumentation for lumbar spinal tuberculosis. World Neurosurg. 2017; 104: 660-667.

11
泌尿生殖系统结核

叶卡捷琳娜·库卡维尼亚,库尔特·G.纳贝尔和
特鲁尔斯·埃里克·比约克朗德·约翰森

概述

泌尿生殖系统结核似乎是一种罕见的疾病,所以它大多被忽视了。泌尿生殖系统结核具有传染性,是不孕不育的原因之一。现代技术使得及时诊断这种感染成为可能,而最佳的治疗可能会挽救患者的器官。

11.1 历史

1894年,波特(Porter)首次提出关于泌尿生殖系统结核的注释[1];这一次,"泌尿生殖系统结核"一词被接受。1937年,威尔德博兹(Wildbolz)[2]提出了泌尿生殖道结核这一术语。虽然没有特别的理由改变这个术语,但医学会批准了新的术语,因为我们有这两个术语。然而,泌尿生殖系统结核一词更准确,因为肾结核通常是原发性的,比生殖器结核更容易被诊断出来。

11.2 定义

泌尿生殖系统结核(urogenital tuberculosis, UGTB)可定义为由结核分枝杆菌(mycobacterium tuberculosis, MTB)或牛分枝杆菌(mycobacterium bovis, M. bovis)引起的任何泌尿生殖器官[肾、尿道和(或)男性或女性生殖器]的感染性炎症。

生殖器结核(genital tuberculosis, GTB)可定义为由结核分枝杆菌或牛

分枝杆菌引起的女性或男性生殖器结核。

尿道结核(urinary tract tuberculosis,UTTB)是上尿路和(或)下尿路的感染性变态反应性炎症,通常继发于肾结核(kidney tuberculosis,KTB),应被认为是KTB的并发症。

本章不包括女性生殖器结核。

11.3 分类

UGTB可分为以下类型:

11.3.1 肾结核

由结核分枝杆菌或牛分枝杆菌引起的肾实质感染性炎症,有4个阶段需要考虑:

阶段1:肾实质结核(非破坏性形式,KTB-1)仅接受保守治疗。KTB-1的损伤很小,没有破坏,通过抗结核药物完全恢复是可能的。静脉尿路造影(intravenous urography,IVU)正常。儿童的尿液分析通常是正常的,但成人可能会发现低水平的白细胞尿。通常情况下,患者没有主诉,常被意外诊断出来。尿液结核分枝杆菌检测是诊断肾结核Ⅰ期的必要方法。

阶段2:结核性乳头炎(小破坏性形式,KTB-2)可以是单侧和双侧、单发和多发。KTB-2应用抗结核药物治疗,但如有并发症,则需行重建手术。并非所有病例都能检测到结核分枝杆菌,细菌可能是耐药的。

阶段3:海绵状肾结核(破坏性形式,KTB-3)。KTB-3的发病机制有两种,一种是从实质结核发病,另一种是从乳头炎发病。第一种方式是在没有连接到集合系统的情况下形成皮质下空洞。皮质下空洞的临床表现类似于肾脓肿,因此通常在手术后做出诊断。第二种方法是破坏乳头,直到形成一个空洞。超过一半的患者会出现并发症。通过抗结核药物完全康复是不可能的,通常需要手术治疗。

阶段4:多发性海绵状肾结核(广泛破坏性形式,KTB-4)。仅用抗结核药物是不可能恢复的,必须进行手术,基本上是肾切除术。

肾结核的并发症包括慢性肾衰竭、瘘管和高血压。

11.3.2 泌尿系结核(UTTB)

尿路结核包括肾盂、输尿管、膀胱和尿道结核。UTTB首先表现为水肿,下一阶段是浸润、溃疡和纤维化。UTTB总是次于KTB。UTTB可细分为以下部分。

11.3.2.1 输尿管结核

输尿管结核通常发生在输尿管的下1/3,但也可能有多处病变。

11.3.2.2 膀胱结核

膀胱结核分为4期[3]:第1期为结节浸润期;第2期为糜烂性溃疡性膀胱炎;第3期为痉挛性膀胱炎;意味着膀胱过度活跃;第4期为膀胱收缩至完全闭塞;前2期为标准抗结核药物治疗,第3期为标准抗结核药物联合氯化曲普铵治疗,第4期为膀胱切除尿流改道或膀胱置换手术。

还有另一种形式的膀胱结核,医源性卡介苗诱导的膀胱结核,它是作为卡介苗治疗膀胱癌的并发症而发展起来的。

11.3.2.3 尿道结核

尿道结核现在并不是一个常见的并发症,通常在狭窄阶段被诊断出来。

11.3.3 男性生殖器结核(MGTB)

男性生殖器结核(male genital tuberculosis,MGTB)分为4类:

11.3.3.1 附睾结核(单侧或双侧)

双侧附睾结核总是继发于前列腺癌。22%的孤立性附睾结核病例常在手术中被意外发现[4]。

11.3.3.2 睾丸结核

睾丸结核总是继发于附睾感染,由于附睾,特别是小叶的广泛供血,附睾感染大多是通过血液传播的。在62%的附睾炎患者中诊断出睾丸结核,每三个患者中就有一个双侧病变。大约12%的睾丸结核病例并发瘘管[4,5]。

11.3.3.3 前列腺结核

前列腺结核是一种经常被忽略的疾病。3/4的前列腺癌男性患者死于各种类型的结核病。但在尸检之前，这一点大多被忽视了[6]。在前列腺结核患者中，79%的合并KTB，31%的合并附睾结核，5%的诊断为孤立性前列腺结核[3-5]。

11.3.3.4 精囊结核

结核性水泡炎继发于前列腺癌，并导致不孕不育。由于干酪样射精液引流困难，精囊结核有钙化倾向。

11.3.3.5 阴茎结核

阴茎结核很少见，但可在与受感染女性发生性交后发生，也可在包皮环切术期间通过阴茎伤口直接感染。阴茎损伤表现为龟头或阴茎皮肤上的溃疡。也可作为卡介苗治疗的一种并发症[8]。

11.3.3.6 泌尿生殖系统结核的并发症

泌尿生殖系统结核的并发症包括狭窄、瘘管、不孕和性功能障碍。

11.3.4 泛发性泌尿生殖系统结核

泛发性泌尿生殖系统结核（generalized urogenital tuberculosis，gUGTB）同时损害肾和泌尿生殖器官；gUGTB一直被认为是一种复杂的结核病形式。

泌尿生殖系统结核的病原学研究。

在分枝杆菌大家族中，结核分枝杆菌和牛分枝杆菌结合在分枝杆菌复合体中，是人类有机体必备的病原体。在80%～95%的UGTB病例中，结核分枝杆菌是由结核分枝杆菌引起的，但由于结核是一种人畜共患感染，牛分枝杆菌也是结核的病原体[9-11]。卡介苗是一种减毒牛分枝杆菌，广泛用于浅表性刀叶癌的治疗。卡介苗治疗可能会并发于医源性卡介苗诱导的UGTB，主要是膀胱或前列腺结核。但在极少数情况下，卡介苗脓毒症已被诊断出来[12-15]。

11.4 诊断

11.4.1 临床特点

UGTB 的临床特征具有非特异性和不稳定性，受多种因素影响。也是延误诊断的原因之一。最常见的主诉是腰部疼痛(高达 80%)和(或)排尿困难(高达 54%)。如果累及尿路，则可能会发生肾绞痛(24%)和肉眼血尿(高达 20%)。前列腺结核表现为会疼痛和排尿困难，半数病例表现为血尿。结核性附睾炎通常始于附睾炎，阴囊器官水肿、肿胀和疼痛是最常见的首发症状。在 68% 的病例中，这种疾病是急性首发的。然而，在 32%～40% 的患者中，这种疾病有一个慢性或无症状的病程[3,16-20]。

11.4.2 体格检查

任何瘘管都要特别注意。阴囊和会阴瘘高度怀疑结核病[18]。在结核性附睾炎急性期，可触及与睾丸紧密连接的坚硬、疼痛、增大的附睾。在慢性病例中，附睾仍然坚硬、增大、无痛，但通常与睾丸边界清楚。在 35%～40% 的病例中，病变发现是双侧的。前列腺结核患者的直肠指诊显示中度增大的结节状前列腺，伴有轻微疼痛[4,5,20]。

11.4.3 实验室检查

应对所有 UGTB 患者进行肺部受累和 HIV 感染筛查。

11.4.3.1 尿液分析和培养试验

90%～100% 的 KTB 患者有白细胞尿，50%～60% 的患者有血尿[3]。在"抗生素时代"之前，无菌脓尿是 KTB 的特殊症状，但现在高达 75% 的患者同时患有非特异性肾盂肾炎和 KTB，因此尿液中可能同时发现尿路病原体和结核分枝杆菌[17-20]。结核分枝杆菌检出对 UGTB 的诊断是绝对肯定的，但近年来只有一半的肺结核患者能检出结核分枝杆菌。因此，对于疑似 UGTB 但无结核分枝杆菌证据的患者，诊断泌尿系结核必须根据其他特征，如皮试、组织学检查、静脉肾盂造影发现空洞、无菌脓尿等[3,21]。

UGTB 的诊断可以通过培养结核分枝杆菌（从适当的临床样本，如尿液、脓液、精液或组织活检）或通过使用快速分子诊断试验（GeneXpert® MTB/RIF）鉴定结核分枝杆菌 DNA 来确认。由于生长速度慢，传统的固体培养系统，包括 Löwenstein-Jensen 斜面或 Middlebrook 7H11 琼脂平板，总是需要 8 周的培养时间才能报告阴性结果。不幸的是，今天标准培养基上的标准培养对 UGTB 患者的效率很低。假阴性结果的主要原因之一是当 UGTB 患者被非特异性 UTI 掩盖时，用阿米卡星和氟喹诺酮类药物治疗时，对 UTI 的经验性治疗不佳。这两种药物对结核分枝杆菌的生长都有负面影响。

有哪些现代技术可以快速识别结核分枝杆菌？首先，分子遗传学方法在结核病诊断中的应用，包括用不同的聚合酶链反应（PCR）技术（FLASH、实时、Hain 生命科学）检测结核分枝杆菌、测定病原体的抗药性（Ⅰ-Ⅱ系列抗结核药物）、鉴定病原体的类型、菌株和从患者分离的分枝杆菌（结核分枝杆菌、非结核分枝杆菌）的基因型。

此外，BACTEC - MGIT - 960 系统，一种全自动、非放射性培养系统，已被推荐用于从临床标本中更快地分离分枝杆菌。每隔 60 min 用氧猝灭荧光传感器技术对培养物进行监测，与传统方法相比，在较短的实验室周转时间内提供了令人满意的性能。因此，BACTEC - MGIT - 960 被广泛认为是诊断结核病的黄金标准。但即使是这种现代的方法也可能给出假阴性的结果。结核分枝杆菌在 BACTEC - MGIT - 960 中的生长可以不被检测到，特别是最具攻击性的北京菌株[3,21]。

11.4.3.2 组织学

活检或手术材料的组织学检查可能会发现上皮样肉芽肿和干酪样坏死，这两种情况很快就会被纤维组织取代，特别是在先前的治疗效果不佳之后。前列腺活检应该在尿道造影后才能进行，以排除空洞[22,23]。

细针吸取细胞学检查（fine-needle aspiration cytology，FNAC）可能有助于诊断男性外生殖器结核[4]。然而，如果临床上包括组织学怀疑肿块是恶性的，应该始终考虑阴囊手术。在未经治疗的 UGTB 活动性患者进行活组织检查后，由于暴发性泛化结核而导致了致命性并发症。

11.4.3.3 影像学

超声检查只能提供泌尿系结核的间接证据。由于79%的病例[24]伴有前列腺癌[24],肾脏超声在"慢性前列腺炎"患者中检测到的病理结果常高度可疑对泌尿生殖系结核。结核性附睾炎和睾丸炎表现为不均匀增大的病灶,可以是均匀的或不均匀,也可以是结节状增大的不均匀低回声病灶[24]。经直肠超声可以显示前列腺的低回声和高回声病变,主要位于周围区域,但也可以显示前列腺结石,这可能是结核炎症的钙化区[24]。

放射学检查对UGTB的早期诊断没有用处。静脉肾盂造影(intravenous pyelography,IVP)适用于有白细胞尿和(或)超声检查异常的患者。所有GTB患者都应该进行逆行尿道造影,以排除前列腺内的空洞。CT提供了更多的信息。在增强CT扫描上,前列腺或精囊结核可见低密度或空洞病变,其原因是坏死和干酪化伴或不伴钙化。如果没有钙化,其结果可能类似于化脓性前列腺脓肿[25,26]。

一般情况下,内窥镜检查及器械干预对UGTB的诊断价值有限。然而,膀胱镜检查适用于所有有排尿困难的UGTB患者。任何黏膜病理都应该进行组织学和细菌学的活检和调查,尽管缺乏特定的发现也并不排除结核的诊断[3]。

11.5 治疗

11.5.1 化学疗法

由于UGTB是一种传染病,应尽快开始抗结核治疗。一旦诊断出活动性结核病,应遵循世卫组织和专家协会指南进行结核病药物治疗[27-31]。

当疾病是早期的,并由药物敏感的结核分枝杆菌引起时,应开出一线抗结核药物。当结核分枝杆菌对一线抗结核药物有耐药性或耐受性差时,会出现严重的不良反应,或者在疾病复发的情况下,都建议使用二线或三线抗结核药物[32]。

11.5.2 抗结核治疗最常见的不良反应

长期接触抗结核药物会增加药物不良反应和毒性的风险。肝很容易受一线抗结核药物的伤害[33]。抗结核药物所致的肝毒性是导致治疗中断的最常见的不良反应。这可能导致病死率、长期发病率升高和治疗依从性降低。高龄和营养状况差（包括基线低蛋白血症）是发生抗结核肝炎的独立预测因子[34]。在另一项研究中，高龄、贫血、耐多药结核病药物、超重/肥胖状况和吸烟史是抗结核药物不良反应的独立危险因素[35]。

利奈唑胺是为数不多的在治疗广泛耐药结核病和多药耐药结核病方面显示出希望的药物之一。长期使用利奈唑胺与毒性有关，如周围和视神经病变。如果患者接受利奈唑胺治疗，糖尿病，特别是在不加控制的情况下，也会导致周围神经病变[35]。

11.5.3　结核病及抗结核治疗对性功能的负面影响

不仅生殖器形式的结核病可能对女性生殖功能产生负面影响。在66%的女性中，肺结核伴有月经异常。然而，在完成抗结核治疗后，76%的月经异常女性恢复了正常的月经周期[36,37]。

抗结核治疗对射精率有不良影响：抗结核治疗2个月后，精子质量下降23.9%，活跃精子数减少10.6%，形态异常精子数减少32.3%[38]。抗结核治疗2个月后，精子质量下降23.9%，活跃精子数减少10.6%，形态异常精子数减少32.3%[38]。为评估性功能，对98例男性肺结核患者进行回顾性研究。分别在抗结核治疗开始前和抗结核治疗3个月后测定阴道内延迟潜伏期。在基线水平上，14.3%的肺结核患者有射精障碍，10.2%的患者早泄，4.1%的患者射精延迟。其余85.7%的患者射精正常[39,40]。经4种抗结核药物（异烟肼、利福平、吡嗪酰胺、链霉素）治疗3个月后，性功能障碍明显改变。射精正常的患者比率下降到61.2%，早泄频率增加了1倍（20.4%），延迟射精的发生率增加了4.5倍（18.4%）[40]。作者强调，男性肺结核患者中射精障碍的比例最初与普通人群相同。他们认为肺结核作为一种疾病并不影响射精功能，但在3个月内用4种药物抗结核治疗，每4个月中就有1/4的患者射精功能明显下降。作者解释说，由于一些抗结核药物的神经毒性，延迟射精的频率增加了4倍。因此，肺结核作为一种疾病不会损害射精功能，但抗结核药物会损害射精功能。未来的研究应该寻找预防这种并发症的方法[40]。在俄罗斯，特别是在西伯利亚，目前有结核病流行[41]。

大约2/3的新诊断患者是年轻男性，性功能和生育能力对他们来说非常重要。对 105 例 18～39 岁初诊肺结核患者的性功能进行了研究[40]。虽然未发现泌尿生殖系统疾病，但肺结核患者从性欲到性高潮的多项指标均有下降。广泛性空洞型肺结核患者的性功能障碍水平明显高于小型性肺结核患者，且这一水平与性功能障碍的严重程度密切相关。

复杂的抗结核化疗影响了肺结核患者的生育力，很可能是通过抑制全身炎症和减少中毒，但即使在治疗 6 个月后，通过有效问卷调查，他们的性功能测试得分也明显下降[60]。

11.5.4 手术治疗

晚期病例需手术治疗，并纠正并发症。最相关的手术干预如表 11-1 所示。

表 11-1 泌尿生殖系统结核的外科治疗

分　类	外　科　治　疗
1. 肾结核	
KTB-3 型，对 2～4 个月的标准疗法耐药（有明显空洞化脓，尿液中有结核分枝杆菌，化脓）耐药	海绵体切除术（肾部分切除术），首选腹腔镜
KTB-4 型	肾切除术，首选腹腔镜
2. 尿路结核	
输尿管、尿道狭窄	标准整形手术
膀胱结核 4 期	膀胱切除术（男性患者为膀胱前列腺切除术），然后进行导管或膀胱置换术
3. 附睾睾丸结核	
有波动感的脓肿	脓肿切开引流术
1～2 个月保守治疗无效，病程缓慢	附睾睾丸切除术
4. 前列腺结核（通常前列腺结核不适合手术）	
脓肿进展	脓肿引流术

所有外科干预均应在抗结核药物覆盖范围内进行。治疗时间由切除组织的组织学检查后决定[42-44]。

11.5.5 结论

结核病至今仍是世界范围内成人感染性疾病的最主要死因。泌尿生殖系统结核起病隐匿、慢性非特异性症状、临床表现隐蔽多变、缺乏临床认识，常被临床漏诊。延误诊断会导致疾病进展、组织和器官损伤以及肾衰竭。UGTB 可表现为慢性尿道炎、血尿、梗阻性尿路病变、不孕症、肾或睾丸肿块，并可导致尿路上皮癌的发生；目前，无菌脓尿在 UGTB 中并不典型。

参考文献

[1] Porter MF III. Uro-genital tuberculosis in the male. Ann Surg. 1894; 20(4): 396-405.
[2] Wildbolz H. Ueber urogenical tuberkulose. Schweiz Med Wochenschr. 1937; 67: 1125.
[3] Kulchavenya E. Urogenital tuberculosis: epidemiology, diagnosis, therapy. Cham/Heidelberg/New York/Dordrecht/London: Springer; 2014. p. 137. ISBN 978-2-319-04836-9. https://doi.org/10.1007/978-3-319-04837-6.
[4] Kulchavenya E, Kim C-S. Male genital tuberculosis. In: Naber KG, Schaeffer AJ, Heyns CF, Matsumoto T, Shoskes DA, Bjerklund Johanses TE, editors. International Consultation on Urogenital Infections. International Consultation on Urological Diseases (ICUD). Arnhem: European Association of Urology (EAU); 2010. p. 892-903. ISBN: 978-90-79754-41-0. http://www.icud.info/urogenitalinfections.html.
[5] Kulchavenya E, Kim CS, Bulanova O, Zhukova I. Male genital tuberculosis: epidemiology and diagnostic. World J Urol. 2012; 30(1): 15-21. Epub 2011 May 21. Review.
[6] Kamyshan IS. Guideline on urogenital tuberculosis. Kiev: Zdorov'e. 2003: 363-424.
[7] Narayana AS, Kelly DG, Duff FA. Tuberculosis of the penis. Br J Urol. 1976; 48(4): 274.
[8] Sharma VK, Sethy PK, Dogra PN, et al. Primary tuberculosis of glans penis after intravesical Bacillus Calmette Guerin immunotherapy. Indian J Dermatol Venereol Leprol. 2011; 77(1): 47-50.
[9] Lewis KE, Lucas MG, Smith R, Harrison NK. Urogenital infection by Mycobacterium bovis relapsing after 50 years. J Infect. 2003; 46(4): 246-248.
[10] de la Rua-Domenech R. Human Mycobacterium bovis infection in the United Kingdom: Incidence, risks, control measures and review of the zoonotic aspects of bovine tuberculosis. Tuberculosis (Edinb). 2006; 86(2): 77-109. Epub 2005 Oct 28.

[11] de Kantor IN, Lobue PA, Thoen CO. Human tuberculosis caused by Mycobacterium bovis in the United States, Latin America and the Caribbean. Int J Tuberc Lung Dis. 2010; 14(11): 1369-1373.

[12] Bhat S, Srinivasa Y, Paul F. Asymptomatic renal BCG granulomatosis: an unusual complication of intravesical BCG therapy for carcinoma urinary bladder. Indian J Urol. 2015; 31 (3): 259-261. https://doi.org/10.4103/0970-1591.156921.

[13] Al-Qaoud T, Brimo F, Aprikian AG, Andonian S. BCG-related renal granulomas managed conservatively: A case series. Can Urol Assoc J. 2015; 9(3-4): E200-203. https://doi.org/10.5489/cuaj.2664.

[14] Pommier JD, Ben Lasfar N, Van Grunderbeeck N, et al. Complications following intravesical bacillus Calmette-Guerin treatment for bladder cancer: a case series of 22 patients. Infect Dis (Lond). 2015; 47(10): 729-735. https://doi.org/10.3109/23744235.2015.1055794. Epub 2015 Jun 16.

[15] Pérez-Jacoiste Asín MA, Fernández-Ruiz M, López-Medrano F, et al. Bacillus Calmette-Guérin (BCG) infection following intravesical BCG administration as adjunctive therapy for bladder cancer: incidence, risk factors, and outcome in a single-institution series and review of the literature. Medicine (Baltimore). 2014; 93(17): 236-254.

[16] Miyake H, Fujisawa M. Tuberculosis in urogenital organs. Nihon Rinsho. 2011; Aug; 69(8): 1417-1421.

[17] Carrillo-Esper R, Moreno-Castañeda L, Hernández-Cruz AE, Aguilar-Zapata D. A renal tuberculosis. Cir Cir. 2010; 78(5): 442-447.

[18] Bennani S, Hafiani M, Debbagh A, el Mrini M, Benjelloun S. Urogenital tuberculosis. Diagnostic aspects. J Urol. 1995; 101(4): 187-190.

[19] Chiang LW, Jacobsen AS, Ong CL, Huang WS. Persistent sterile pyuria in children? Don't forget tuberculosis! Singap Med J. 2010; 51(3): 48-50.

[20] Hoang NPC, Nhan LVH, Le Chuyen V. Genitourinary tuberculosis: diagnosis and treatment. Urology. 2009; (Supplement 4A): S241.

[21] Hemal AK, Gupta NP, Rajeev TP, Kumar R, Dar L, Seth P. Polymerase chain reaction in clinically suspected genitourinary tuberculosis: comparison with intravenous urography, bladder biopsy, and urine acid fast bacilli culture. Urology. 2000; 56(4): 570-574.

[22] Kulchavenya EV, Brizhatyuk EV, Baranchukova AA, Cherednichenko AG, Klimova IP. Diagnostic Algorithm for prostate tuberculosis. Tuberk I bolezn legk. 2014; 5: 10-15.

[23] Stasinou T, Bourdoumis A, Owegie P, Kachrilas S, Buchholz N, Masood J. Calcification of the vas deferens and seminal vesicles: a review. Can J Urol. 2015; 22(1): 7594-7598.

[24] Turkvatan A, Kelahmet E, Yazgan C, Olcer T. Sonographic findings in tuberculous epididymo-orchitis. J Clin Ultrasound. 2004; 32(6): 302-305.

[25] Wang LJ, Wong YC, Chen CJ, Lim KE. CT features of genitourinary tuberculosis. J Comput Assist Tomogr. 1997; 21(2): 254-258.

[26] Wang JH, Sheu MH, Lee RC. Tuberculosis of the prostate: MR appearance. J

Comput Assist Tomogr. 1997; 21(4): 639-640.
[27] British Thoracic Society. Guidelines for the prevention and management of Mycobacterium tuberculosis infection and disease in adult patients with chronic kidney disease BTS Guideline Group on behalf of The British Thoracic Society Standards of Care Committee and Joint Tuberculosis Committee. Thorax. 2010; 65: 559-570. https://doi.org/10.1136/thx.2009.133173.
[28] O'Donnell R. Drugs in renal failure. Antituberculous drugs. South West Medicines Information. NHS Ref: dosage adjustment of anti tuberculosis medication in patients with Renal Failure Department of Internal Medicine, PMHC.
[29] Sharma JB, Singh N, Dharmendra S, Singh UB, P V, Kumar S, Roy KK, Hari S, Iyer V, Sharma SK. Six months versus nine months anti-tuberculous therapy for female genital tuberculosis: a randomized controlled trial. Eur J Obstet Gynecol Reprod Biol. 2016; 203: 264-273.
[30] Chang CH, Chen YF, Wu VC, Shu CC, Lee CH, Wang JY, Lee LN, Yu CJ. Acute kidney injury due to anti-tuberculosis drugs: a five-year experience in an aging population. BMC Infect Dis. 2014; 14: 23.
[31] WHO Guidelines for the treatment of drug-susceptible tuberculosis and patient care. 2017 update. WHO/HTM/TB/2017. 05 http://apps.who.int/iris/bitstream/10665/255052/1/9789241550000-eng.pdf?ua=1. Accessed 30 Nov 2017.
[32] Kulchavenya E. Current therapy and surgery for urogenital tuberculosis: Springer International Publishing Switzerland, 2016; ISBN 978-3-319-28288-6; ISBN 978-3-319-28290-9 (eBook); https://doi.org/10.1007/978-3319-28290-9: 97 pages.
[33] Singla R, Sharma SK, Mohan A, Makharia G, Sreenivas V, Jha B, et al. Evaluation of risk factors for antituberculosis treatment induced hepatotoxicity. Indian J Med Res. 2010; 132: 81-86.
[34] Chung-Delgado K, Revilla-Montag A, Guillen-Bravo S, Velez-Segovia E, Soria-Montoya A, Nuñez-Garbin A, et al. Factors associated with anti-tuberculosis medication adverse effects: a case-control study in Lima, Peru. PLoS One. 2011; 6(11): e27610. https://doi.org/10.1371/journal.pone.0027610. Epub 2011 Nov 16.
[35] Swaminathan A, du Cros P, Seddon JA, Mirgayosieva S, Asladdin R, Dusmatova Z. Peripheral neuropathy in a diabetic child treated with linezolid for multidrug-resistant tuberculosis: a case report and review of the literature. BMC Infect Dis. 2017; 17(1): 417. https://doi.org/10.1186/s12879-017-2499-1.
[36] Hassan WA, Darwish AM. Impact of pulmonary tuberculosis on menstrual pattern and fertility. Clin Respir J. 2010; 4(3): 157-161. https://doi.org/10.1111/j.1752-699X.2009.00166.x.
[37] Hassan WA, Darwish AM. Impact of pulmonary tuberculosis on menstrual pattern and fertility. Chest. 2009; 136(1): 326. https://doi.org/10.1378/chest.09-0594.
[38] Kulchavenya EV, Osadchii AV. The role of pathogenetic therapy in preserving ejaculate fertility in patients with tuberculosis of prostate. Urologiia. 2016; 3: 14-18.

[39] Kulchavenya E, Medvedev S. Therapy for pulmonary tuberculosis as a reason for ejaculatory disorders. J Sex Med. 2011; 8(suppl 5): 384-405 - HP-23.

[40] Kulchavenya E, Scherban M, Brizhatyuk E, Osadchiy A. Sexual dysfunction in male patients with pulmonary tuberculosis. J Microbiol Infect Dis. 2012; 2(3): 124-126. https://doi.org/10.5799/ahinjs.02.2012.03.0057.

[41] Kulchavenya E, Zhukova I, Kholtobin D. Spectrum of urogenital tuberculosis. J Infect Chemother. 2013; 19(5): 880-883.

[42] Kholtobin D, Kulchavenya EV. Surgery for bladder tuberculosis. Palmarium Academium Publishing (Germany); 2013. p. 76.

[43] Singh V, Sinha RJ, Sankhwar SN, Sinha SM. Reconstructive surgery for tuberculous contracted bladder: experience of a center in northern India. Int Urol Nephrol. 2011; Jun; 43(2): 423-430.

[44] Suárez-Grau JM, Bellido-Luque JA, Pastrana-Mejía A, et al. Laparoscopic surgery of an enterovesical fistula of tuberculous origin (terminal ileum and sigmoid colon). Rev Esp Enferm Dig. 2012; 104(7): 391-392.

12
心血管结核

哈利勒·法提赫·阿斯根和巴林·基里尔马兹

12.1 概论

结核病在发达国家并不常见,但它仍然是地方病,在非洲和亚洲的一些地区经常出现。此外,免疫功能受损的患者,特别是 HIV 患者的数目增加,亦是结核病及其并发症增加的原因。根据世界卫生组织(WHO)的数据,今天世界上 1/3 的人口感染了结核病,它是感染性疾病患者中最常见的死亡原因[31]。

EPTB 通常见于胸膜、淋巴结、腹部和中枢神经系统[35]。1%~2%的结核病患者涉及心血管系统[4,27,30,33,35,50]。尸检中心脏结核的发病率约为 0.25%[33]。已有研究表明,死于结核病的患者心脏受累率约为 2%[43]。只有 0.5%的 EPTB 患者有心脏受累,而且更多见于免疫功能低下的患者[53]。主要受累部位是心包[35,50,53]。其他形式的心血管受累包括心内膜、心肌、瓣膜或冠状动脉,动脉炎和动脉瘤极为罕见[27]。结核累及心肌可能导致心律失常、心脏性猝死、充血性心力衰竭和动脉瘤。此外,大动脉炎可能导致霉菌性动脉瘤、假性动脉瘤和破裂[43]。

12.2 结核性心包炎

心包是肺结核最常累及的心脏组织。不到 1%的结核病患者出现心包炎[23,40]。一般来说,10%~11%的心包炎患者有结核病病因[23,57]。结核性心包炎在流行地区发病率较高,据报道在发展中国家占心包炎患者的 40%~70%[40,43,50]。相比之下,在发达国家,只有 4%的心包炎患者有结核病病因[40,43]。此外,它的发病率在 HIV 流行的地区更高[40,57]。

12.2.1 病理学

结核性心包炎总是与位于身体任何部位的心外感染病灶相关[50]。它通过3条主要途径扩散到心包：淋巴扩散（从气管旁、支气管周围和纵隔淋巴结）；血源性扩散（主要发生在免疫功能低下的患者中）；或者很少直接从邻近结构（肺、胸膜和脊柱）扩散[40,43,50]。淋巴和血行播散是主要途径。本病的病理生理分为4个阶段：① 纤维蛋白渗出伴多形核浸润伴较高数量的分枝杆菌；② 浆液性或浆液性渗出伴淋巴细胞浸润（单核细胞和泡沫细胞）；③ 渗液吸收导致干酪性肉芽肿，心包因纤维蛋白和胶原沉积及纤维化而增厚；④ 瘢痕狭窄伴广泛钙化[9,38,40]。内脏和壁心包的纤维化、粘连和钙化形成一个坚硬而收缩的纤维钙化包膜包裹心脏，在缩窄性心包炎阶段限制舒张期充盈和最终收缩期射血[40]。

结核性心包炎是一种典型的少菌性疾病[43]。结核分枝杆菌的蛋白质依附于心包，可触发辅助性T细胞亚型1（TH-1）淋巴细胞介导的超敏反应，刺激细胞因子的释放[9,40,43]。细胞因子释放激活巨噬细胞，诱导心包炎症和肉芽肿形成，从而导致渗出性渗出和后遗症[40,43]。结核性心包积液的患者有细胞因子谱（肿瘤坏死因子α以及白细胞介素1和2），干扰素-γ的产生增加，这表明发生了由TH-1淋巴细胞协调的超敏反应[9,40]。最常涉及的细胞因子是肿瘤坏死因子-α[57]。细胞因子也可能导致发热、体重减轻和虚弱[57]。引起细胞溶解的抗肌膜抗体可能在渗出性心包炎中起作用[40]。

12.2.2 临床特点

虽然病程大多是隐匿的，并进展为慢性缩窄性心包炎，但也可以看到与心包填塞有关的急性和暴发性图片[7,15]。填塞被认为是结核性心包炎的急性并发症，而缩窄性心包炎是慢性并发症[43]。临床表现高度多变，包括急性心包炎伴或不伴积液、心脏压塞、慢性心包积液、急性缩窄性心包炎、亚急性缩窄性心包炎、渗出性缩窄性心包炎或慢性缩窄性心包炎，以及心包钙化[37,50]。它通常表现为4种临床症状之一：急性心包炎、渗出性心包炎、肌包炎或缩窄性心包炎[43]。这种疾病的常见表现是心包积液、缩窄性心包炎或积液和缩窄性心包炎[40]。这种疾病可能在免疫功能低下的患者（HIV

等)中进展得更有侵略性;包括呼吸困难、血流动力学不稳定和心肌受累在内的临床表现往往更严重[43]。

12.2.2.1 结核性心包炎和心包积液

这种疾病的发病大多是潜伏的[7,15,40]。它通常表现为"慢性进行性发热病"[7]。结核性心包炎患者一般有体重减轻、咳嗽、呼吸困难、矫形呼吸、胸痛、盗汗、发热、心动过速、心脏肿大和胸腔积液[7,23,40,51,57]。最常见的症状是咳嗽、呼吸困难和发热[7,40]。胸痛相对较少见[7,43]。患者常有窦性心动过速、反常脉搏(>12 mmHg)、中心静脉压升高、心尖冲动明显、心音低沉、心包摩擦、肝大、腹水、外周水肿等充血性心力衰竭症状[7,15,40,43,51,57]。右上腹疼痛可能是由于肝充血[40]。影响颈腺的外周淋巴结病变已有报道[7]。典型的急性心包炎三联症,包括胸痛、摩擦和心电图改变并不常见,仅见于3%～8%的结核性心包炎患者[43]。如果心包积液迅速或代偿机制不充分,可能会发生低血压和压塞[43]。10%的结核性心包积液患者有心脏压塞[40]。结核性心包积液的特点是渗出性的,它含有高蛋白和白细胞计数增加,主要包括淋巴细胞和单核细胞,并且经常出血[40]。大约一半的患者没有肺部病变的证据[23]。

结核性心包炎可能累及下层心肌。心肌损伤生物标志物(肌钙蛋白、肌酸激酶等)水平升高,与心肌损伤相关的心电图改变,以及左心室收缩功能受损,可能与结核性心包炎的存在有关[43]。

12.2.2.2 缩窄性心包炎

尽管抗结核药物和皮质类固醇治疗得当,30%～60%的结核性心包积液患者仍会发生缩窄性心包炎[9,40]。它被认为是结核病最重要的并发症之一。在发展中国家,缩窄性心包炎最常见的原因是结核病,报告发病率为38%～83%[9]。入院时因结核性心包炎而出现的压塞被发现与随后缩窄性心包炎的发展相关[57]。

壁层心包和脏层心包由于心包炎引起的纤维化或纤维蛋白渗出而增厚和融合[9]。由于弗兰克-斯塔林定律,这种情况在心周围形成了一层坚硬的皮肤,限制了心室的舒张期充盈,并最终减少了心的每搏量。心室不能容纳和泵出足够数量的血液会导致充血性心力衰竭[9]。长期的狭窄可能导致心肌纤维化和萎缩,出现心力衰竭,使手术结果恶化[9]。

临床表现可能从无症状到严重的挛缩[40]。它可以从急性心包炎进展到收缩期，经过渗出期和吸收期，也可以表现为无急性心包炎病史的心包狭窄[9]。心包敲击，一种早期的舒张期声音，由收缩的左心室迅速充盈引起，听诊时可听到第二心音的分裂。心电图上可见低电压复合波和心房颤动，X线片上可见心胸比率增大[40]。

虽然结核性心包炎在免疫功能低下的患者中可能具有更具侵袭性的临床特征，但据报道，与HIV阴性患者相比，HIV阳性患者缩窄性心包炎的发生率明显较低[9]。因为结核性心包炎和随后的纤维化和肉芽肿的形成主要由TH-1细胞调控，HIV感染的存在降低了对结核分枝杆菌蛋白的过敏反应和炎症过程[9]。

12.2.2.3 渗出性缩窄性心包炎

渗出性缩窄性心包炎（effusive-constrictive pericarditis，ECP）是一种罕见的结核表现，由内脏心包收缩和压迫性心包积液引起[45]。它可能发生在从心包积液到缩窄性心包炎的连续期间[45]。ECP的患病率为4%～4.5%[45]。60%的ECP病例的病因是结核病[45]。积液和内脏心包收缩都会增加心包周围的压力[40]。ECP的治疗比较困难。心包穿刺术不能减轻心包压力，损害心脏的舒张充盈，因为增厚的心包层之间的纤维素性心包带严格地使心包积液形成房室状，阻止了心包积液的完全引流[40,45]，因此心包穿刺术不能缓解心包压力，损害心的舒张期充盈[40,45]。此外，由于内脏收缩，心包穿刺后心包压力仍然升高[40]。尽管心包内压降至接近0 mmHg，但心包穿刺后右心房压力持续升高提示ECP[45]。同样，这些患者的心包切除术效果通常有限，因为几乎不可能去除包裹在内脏心包的纤维蛋白渗出物[40]。这些患者可以进行内脏心包切除术来治疗持续性心力衰竭[45]。病死率为4%～50%[45]。

12.2.3 诊断

胸片、心电图和超声心动图在结核性心包炎的诊断和治疗中是必不可少的[43]。胸部X线片显示90%以上的病例心脏轮廓增大[40]。它还可能显示肺结核和胸腔积液的放射学证据[7]。在结核性心包炎患者中可以看到心电图的改变，包括非特异性ST-T改变、QRS波群微电压、电交替和心房颤动[35,40]。心电图上微电压的出现通常与心包积液有关[40]。超声心动图是诊断心包积液和心包狭窄的一种准确、无创的方法,但不能提示病因。结核性心包炎常见心包积液,心包各层间有纤维蛋白束和心包增厚,但不具特异性[7,40,51]。在缩窄性心包炎中,超声心动图可以看到心包囊或心脏周围厚厚的皮肤中有厚厚的纤维蛋白渗出,这会减少心脏的运动[40]。另外,CT扫描或MRI可以用来确定心包积液、心包增厚和纵隔淋巴结的存在[7]。几乎所有的结核性心包炎患者都可以检测到纵隔淋巴结病变,而抗结核治疗使其消退或消失,这提示了结核病的病因[7,51]。通常肿大的淋巴结分别是主肺淋巴结(63%)、气管旁淋巴结(52%)、隆突淋巴结(41%)、气管前淋巴结(26%)和肺门淋巴结(15%)[7]。镓-67和铟-111核素显像可用于结核性心包炎的诊断,但其结果不能揭示结核病的病因[7]。因为证明心包炎患者的另一个器官中存在结核是结核性心包炎的高度提示,肺结核病或心外结核的存在应该通过培养和其他技术来探索[7,37]。结核菌素皮肤试验由于其高度的假阴性(25%~33%)和假阳性(30%~40%)结果而不能用于诊断[37,51,57]。检测结果为阴性并不排除结核病,但是,如果检测结果呈强阳性,应该会增加对结核病病因学的怀疑[51]。应在痰中寻找抗酸杆菌,但是只有10%~55%的患者呈阳性[40]。如果痰和心包液检查结果不确定,洗胃、尿培养和右斜角淋巴结活检可以用来识别抗酸杆菌的存在[7,40]。

　　明确的诊断主要是通过对心包液和组织进行微生物学和病理学检查,以显示结核杆菌或肉芽肿[7,43]。所有疑似结核性心包炎的患者都应该进行心包穿刺术[40]。通常建议进行心包活检以获取心包组织样本[57]。这两种手术都可以通过适当的心包切开术同时进行。这种方法还可以引流心包积液进行治疗,并防止心包积液再积聚[57]。这两种手术都可以通过适当的心包切开术同时进行。这种方法还可以引流心包积液进行治疗,并防止心包积液再积聚[57]。需要鉴定心包液或组织样本中的结核分枝杆菌,以及鉴定组织中的干酪性肉芽肿[37]。心包液培养比心包液涂片和心包组织学更能提示结核病病因的诊断[7,40,51],但是分离或鉴定干酪性肉芽肿往往很困难。直接涂片检查只有0~42%的患者心包液中检测到结核杆菌,培养法检测到53%~75%的患者心包液中有结核杆菌[40]。此外,这不是一种及时的方法,可能会导致诊断的延误[57]。心包活检的诊断价值约为10%~64%[40,51]。它提供的阳性结果比心包液样本更频繁,应该进行[15,57]。但是要记住,心包液和心包组织检查的正常结果并不能排除结核性心包炎。

为提高结核性心包炎的诊断水平,提出了结核病流行地区的预测模型[51]。评分系统有 5 个临床和实验室变量:盗汗 1 分,体重减轻 1 分,发热 $>38℃$ 2 分,白细胞计数 $<10×10^9/L$ 3 分,血清球蛋白 $>40 g/L$ 3 分。结果表明,可疑心包炎患者总分 $\geqslant 6$ 分,诊断结核性心包炎的敏感性为 86%,特异性为 84%[51]。

传统的诊断工具不足以诊断结核性心包炎[51],可以使用新的技术,包括聚合酶链反应方法来识别结核分枝杆菌,酶联免疫斑点试验检测结核分枝杆菌抗原特异性 T 细胞,腺苷脱氨酶活性,心包溶菌酶,以及结核性心包积液中干扰素-γ 浓度[37,40,43,51]。它们为结核性心包炎的诊断提供了快速而准确的结果。通过 PCR 方法在心周液和组织样本中鉴定出属于结核分枝杆菌的遗传物质[7]。它的诊断准确率接近传统的微生物学和病理学方法[7]。该方法对组织样本的灵敏度(80%)高于对液体的灵敏度(15%)[7,40,51]。虽然它比培养法更快地提供结果,但高污染率和假阳性结果(灵敏度 32%)使 PCR 不适合日常临床实践[7,40,51]。结果表明,心包 ADA 值升高($\geqslant 35 U/L$)和干扰素-γ 水平升高($>200 pg/L$)对诊断结核性心包炎具有较高的敏感性($>90\%$)和特异性($>70\%$)[7,40]。肾上腺皮质激素水平与 T 细胞活性有关[7]。对于 ADA 水平较高的患者,应排除细菌性心包炎和肿瘤疾病[51]。干扰素-γ 被推荐为一种更具提示性的方法[51]。

12.2.4 治疗

结核性心包炎的治疗包括立即联合药物治疗,疗程不同(6 个月、9 个月、12 个月)[37,38]。治疗的目的既是为了治疗急性压塞症状,又是为了防止缩窄性心包炎的发生[57]。抗结核治疗显著提高了存活率,死亡率已从抗生素前的 80%~90% 下降到目前 HIV 阴性患者的 8%~17% 和 HIV 阳性患者的 17%~34%,但并不能阻止缩窄性心包炎的发展[40]。对于 EPTB,建议采用利福平、异烟肼、吡嗪酰胺和乙胺丁醇至少 2 个月,然后是异烟肼和利福平共 6 个月的联合药物治疗[40]。类固醇可与抗结核联合治疗以降低病死率、症状严重程度、复发和再住院率、缩窄性心包炎的发生率以及心包穿刺或心包切除术的必要性[15,37,43]。但辅助使用类固醇仍然存在争议,因为一些作者已经证明它们不能降低病死率或不需要心包切除术[15,43,57]。

开放手术引流与心包穿刺是治疗结核性心包炎的另一个有争议的问

题[57]。一些作者推荐对结核性心包炎进行早期手术,包括完全开放引流,以防止反复心包穿刺和慢性缩窄性心包炎的发展[15,38,40,57]。在此过程中有机会获得心包活检也有利于开放引流[57]。一般说来,尽管有或没有反复渴望或有心包增厚和收缩的药物治疗,心包积液仍持续存在的患者需要手术治疗[30]。在未经治疗的患者中,结核性心包炎的病死率可能高达85%[37]。据报道,未经特殊治疗的患者平均生存期为3.7个月[7]。

缩窄性心包炎的治疗包括6个月的抗结核药物和心包切除术[40,43]。关于心包切除术的时机尚有争议。虽然一些作者建议所有缩窄性心包炎患者立即手术,但另一些作者建议对内科治疗失败的患者立即手术[40]。在后一种建议中,如果患者有心包钙化(慢性病的后遗症),手术不应推迟[40]。中心静脉压一般在术后2~4天下降,术后4周恢复正常[9],但是大约一半的患者在心包切除术后左心室舒张充盈异常,这是由心肌纤维化和萎缩或不完全去皮质引起的[9]。心包切除术的手术死亡率为3%~16%,在有广泛钙化和粘连的患者中可高达19%[9,40,43]。心包切除术后可能会出现急性心脏扩张和衰竭,这主要是由于心肌萎缩的发生[9]。可以观察到心包切除术后由于心室扩张或乳头肌延长而发生或加重的二尖瓣和三尖瓣反流[9]。

12.3 心肌结核

1664年,土耳其医师毛罗科达特(Maurocordat)首次报道了心肌结核[35]。虽然结核主要累及心包,但心肌很少受到影响[50]。结核分枝杆菌对心包的亲和力比对心肌的亲和力高的原因尚不清楚[27]。心肌结核多发生于心包疾病[41]。孤立性心肌结核极为罕见,患病率为0.2%~2%[23,41,43,50]。结核累及冠状动脉和心内膜的情况极为罕见,通常与心脏其他部位的感染有关[23,50]。心肌结核通常是死后诊断的,在所有尸检中发病率<0.3%[35,50,54]。

12.3.1 病理学

感染通过直接侵犯心包或肺腔、血行播散或逆行淋巴播散到达心肌[35,41,43,50]。感染的源头是肺部[35]。受累类型有3种:① 以中央型为特征的结节(结核球);② 血行播散所致的粟粒型结节;③ 弥漫性浸润,伴富含淋巴细胞和巨细胞的结核性心包炎[4,12,23,27,35,41,43]。可以看到心内膜粟粒型结节、多倍体结节、瓣膜上的结核结节和含有包裹的结核杆菌的血栓[23]。最常受影响的心腔是左心室(68%)。它可导致二尖瓣和三尖瓣关闭不全,但瓣膜狭窄和半月瓣受累并不常见[41]。

12.3.2 临床特点

心肌结核患者通常没有症状[27,41]。与心包炎不同,心肌结核会引起心肌炎,从而导致严重的并发症,包括心律失常和心力衰竭[53]。有症状的患者可有房室性心动过速、室颤、传导缺陷、长QT综合征、充血性心力衰竭、扩张型心肌病、室壁瘤和假性壁瘤、上腔静脉阻塞、右心室阻塞、瓣膜功能不全、冠状动脉炎,甚至心脏性猝死[2,4,5,13,18,21,27,33,35,41,43,54]。伴有心包受累导致渗出、粘连或狭窄会使心肌结核的症状复杂化[54]。抗结核药物的使用可能导致心律失常,包括异烟肼和莫西沙星引起的QT间期延长和尖端扭动[35]。

12.3.3 诊断

心肌结核的诊断通常在尸检时做出[41]。应该在有结核暴露史或地方病流行区出现非缺血性心律失常、充血性心力衰竭或心源性休克的患者中考虑这种情况[27,41,42]。据报道,心脏MRI和晚期钆强化可以描述心脏结核瘤和心肌浸润[27]。如果临床怀疑强烈,影像学提示结核病因,心内膜心肌活检是早期诊断的指标[12,27]。

12.3.4 治疗

关于死前病例的治疗知识有限,基本上依赖于经验指导[27]。标准的4种药物抗结核治疗用于治疗心肌结核及其并发症[41,43]。治疗的持续时间尚不清楚。β-受体阻滞剂可用于治疗室性心律失常,但尚未在该适应证中得到验证[27]。辅助性类固醇的功效也存在争议[27]。

12.4 主动脉结核和动脉瘤

继发于结核感染的真菌性主动脉动脉瘤首先由卡门(Kamen)于1895

年描述[8,39,60]。这是一个非常罕见且危及生命的实体[3,28,36,39,49,60]。有关该病的文献知识主要基于病例报告[8,39]。在帕克赫斯特（Parkhurst）和德克尔（Decker）的报告[48]中，1902年至1951年在22 792例自体中发现的338例主动脉瘤中，仅有1例（0.3%）发现结核性主动脉瘤。这份报告属于前抗生素时代，可以假设，由于抗结核药物的使用，今天继发于结核病感染的主动脉瘤的发病率要少得多[20]。潜伏性肺结核患者中有1%的人患有结核性大动脉炎[3]。免疫功能低下的患者患主动脉炎和动脉瘤的风险很高[36]。虽然在抗生素前时代（1950年之前）发表的病例报告大多来自身体解剖，但最近几年发表的报告表明，由于改进了成像和手术方法，这种疾病的最终诊断和成功治疗已经成为可能[8,22]。

12.4.1 病理学

结核性主动脉瘤在腹主动脉和胸主动脉中的出现频率相同[3,8,36,39,43]。它不常累及周围动脉，包括锁骨下动脉、颈动脉、髂总动脉、肝、肾、股动脉和无名动脉[3,14,16,39]。结核感染通过2条途径到达主动脉：① 通常（在75%的患者中）直接从邻近的传染性病变如纵隔淋巴结炎（63%）、肺部病变、脓胸、心包炎、脊柱炎或椎旁脓肿侵入，以及② 罕见的血源性或淋巴管炎从原发病变扩散[8,14,16,20,22,28,32,36,39,46,47,49,60]。与升主动脉相比，降主动脉更容易感染结核病，46%的结核病主动脉瘤位于降主动脉，而升主动脉只有10%左右[8,14,28,49]。这种倾向可以通过降主动脉靠近纵隔淋巴结来解释[8,14,49]。位于主动脉弓远端和左肺韧带的两组特定的纵隔淋巴结是主动脉弓远端和膈上主动脉的直接感染和动脉瘤的罪魁祸首[46]。肾下段是腹主动脉最常见的受累部位[36]。

主动脉感染与主动脉狭窄、霉菌性动脉瘤、假性动脉瘤或自身免疫性主动脉炎相关[8]。描述了4种类型的结核累及动脉系统：① 内膜的粟粒性感染；② 附着于内膜的结核性息肉；③ 多层动脉壁的感染；④ 动脉瘤的形成[8,22,47]。此外，最近还描述了一种狭窄型主动脉结核[8]。它可能是对结核抗原超敏反应的结果[36]。涉及主动脉（获得性狭窄）或肾动脉的狭窄病变可导致高血压[43,49]。直接血源性扩散可引起主动脉内膜感染，但经血管或淋巴管侵犯可将感染扩展至中膜或外膜[22,32,36,39,47]。结核杆菌也可能寄宿在动脉粥样斑块中，改变血管壁对感染的抵抗力，并通过主动脉壁传播[8,32,36]。

主动脉壁感染导致组织破坏和坏死[16,39]。主动脉壁破坏后扩张形成真正的动脉瘤，称为霉菌性动脉瘤。另一方面，如果坏死累及整个主动脉壁，它可能破裂，导致大量出血或形成血管周围血肿[3,16,22]。包膜血肿的吸收和残腔与主动脉腔的连通会产生假性动脉瘤[16,39]。与真正的动脉瘤相比，假性动脉瘤没有动脉壁的全部三层，这导致动脉瘤破裂和致命出血的倾向，并且通常是囊状的[60]。通常，所有结核性主动脉瘤都没有钙化[8]。大多数结核动脉瘤是孤立的、假性的和球状的，有很高的破裂和致命出血的风险[8,14,20,22,36]。肺结核病血管受累的另一个典型表现是 Rasmussen 动脉瘤，这是一种动脉炎，发生在靠近空洞的血管上，导致这些患者反复咯血[55,60]。

非结核分枝杆菌包括卡介苗，一种用于膀胱癌或黑色素瘤辅助免疫治疗的牛分枝杆菌减毒株，以及鸟分枝杆菌-细胞内分枝杆菌也被报道会导致主动脉瘤和假性动脉瘤[3,39]。

12.4.2 临床特点

该病的临床表现从无症状到破裂、出血和休克。结核性主动脉瘤患者年龄 6~86 岁，平均（50±16）岁。两性平等参与[36]。根据动脉瘤的部位，患者有发热、体重减轻、搏动性或可触及的肿块、胸痛、吞咽困难、声音嘶哑、嘶哑、咯血、肠出血、瘘管、腹痛或背痛[8,14,16,20,22,28,43]。患者通常有 3 种临床表现：① 持续性胸痛、背痛或腹痛；② 大出血或休克；③ 可触及或搏动性肿块迅速扩大[36]。动脉瘤破裂与高病死率有关。已有食管、空肠、胃、肺树、腹腔、十二指肠和结肠破裂的报道[3]。可以看到急性主动脉综合征，包括主动脉夹层[49]。升主动脉的动脉瘤可能延伸到主动脉根部和 Valsalva 窦，并可能导致主动脉瓣关闭不全和心脏压塞[43,47]。最常见的死亡原因是破裂并大出血、粟粒型肺结核和充血性心力衰竭[36]。

12.4.3 诊断

诊断是困难的，应该尽早确定，以防止破裂和相关的死亡[49]。活动性结核的存在或既往病史有助于指导临床医师进行这一具有挑战性的诊断。建议 CT 和 MRI 检查主动脉和动脉瘤[16,22,36]。主动脉壁增厚可能是无病因的大动脉炎[49]。在这种情况下，MRI 更敏感[49]。成像过程中出现对比剂外渗提示动脉瘤破裂，是急诊手术的指征[43]。主动脉造影以前是主要的诊断工具，但它已经被超声、CT 和 MRI 所取代，它们可以方便地以非侵入性的方式检测动脉瘤[16,20]。另外，结核动脉瘤在血管造影中可能没有充盈缺损[36]。

手术标本的组织学检查显示肉芽肿性主动脉炎有干酪性坏死，且 Ziehl-Neelsen 染色抗酸杆菌阳性[49]，最终可确定诊断。检测结果为阴性并不排除结核病病因的诊断。

12.4.4 治疗

单纯的内科或外科治疗都不足以完全治愈。最佳治疗方法是术前、术后联合应用抗结核药物和手术方法[8,14,16,20,22,32,36]。结核病动脉瘤一旦确诊，应立即开始 4 种药物治疗，覆盖术后时间，并紧急手术[8,14,22,36,47]。抗结核治疗的持续时间存在争议，但对于有严重全身感染的患者，抗结核治疗应该延长到至少 9~12 个月[3]。一些作者建议假体植入后终生使用抗生素治疗[3]。对于解剖外搭桥术的患者，应首选延长抗生素治疗，以防止因复发感染而导致的主动脉残端爆裂[3]。

手术选择包括解剖外搭桥、主动脉导管原位植入、补片闭合或直接闭合主动脉瓣，以及腔内动脉瘤修补术[3,8,22,60]。动脉瘤的大小不是手术需要的限制，因为即使是直径降到 1 cm 的小假性动脉瘤也可能破裂并导致致命出血[22,36]。切除受感染的主动脉段及其周围组织，并结合动脉重建下体血运是此类病例中常见的手术方式[20,32,60]。主动脉壁切除的范围应通过肉眼观察来决定，而不是耗时的冰冻切片和组织学检查，以缩短与夹闭相关的缺血时间[8,22]。含有感染性物质的边缘切除不充分与复发有关[8]。根据瓣膜大小选择主动脉修复术的类型：在存在较大瓣膜的情况下应插入间置移植物；否则可进行补片修补[8]。通常，重建真性动脉瘤需要间置移植物，但假性动脉瘤可以进行补片或直接闭合[20]。在存在活动性感染或脓肿形成的情况下，完全切除动脉瘤并扩大切除感染组织之后，应进行解剖外搭桥手术，使假体材料远离感染区[20]。动脉瘤复发和移植物感染可能发生[60]。术前抗结核药物和辅助措施，如椎旁脓肿引流和抗生素浸泡的植骨，可能有助于预防感染的持续或复发[10,16,20]。需要密切的术后随访以发现复发[20,22]。

手术死亡率为14%~20%,急诊手术死亡率高达50%[3,60]。围手术期死亡的原因是消化道大出血、主动脉肠瘘、肾衰竭、另一个结核性动脉瘤破裂和急性心力衰竭[16]。

目前,结核动脉瘤的血管内治疗日益成为首选方法[14]。在血管内治疗中,清创和移除感染组织是手术成功的主要部分是不可能的[14]。在持续感染的情况下,药物治疗的有效性降低,破裂和致命出血的风险增加[14]。因此,仔细选择患者是支架移植治疗成功的关键因素[10]。据报道,放置血管内假体治疗结核动脉瘤有很高的感染、复发和出血风险[39]。在手术过程中相对无菌的患者有更好的结果和更低的长期并发症[10]。此外,血管内治疗可以被认为是通向手术的桥梁,或者是姑息性的目的治疗[32]。

12.5 多发性大动脉炎(高安综合征)

大动脉炎(takayasu arteritis,TA)是一种罕见的原因不明的大血管血管炎,主要累及主动脉及其主要分支,包括锁骨下动脉和颈动脉。它主要是一种炎症性疾病,引起慢性进行性血管壁炎症,原因是血管壁向心性增厚,导致动脉狭窄,并伴有缺血性并发症或动脉瘤形成[26]。TA的临床表现与全身炎症和血管病变部位有关。全身炎症会导致身体症状,包括发热、不适、盗汗、食欲缺乏、关节痛和淋巴结病,而血管并发症包括脉搏缺陷、跛行、头晕、视力障碍、杂音和手臂之间的血压差[34]。

半个多世纪以来,人们一直建议考虑结核病和TA之间存在联系[19,55,58,59]。两个未经证实致病机制的临床实体之间存在临床相关性[26]。与普通人群相比,TA患者的结核病患病率更高[19,34,59]。来自亚洲、南美和非洲的病例系列显示,TA患者的结核病发病率介于22%~70%,而这些地区普通人群的结核病发病率为0.03%~1.5%[19,59]。纯化蛋白衍生物(purified protein derivative,PPD)在81%~100%的TA患者中呈阳性,而在正常对照中为66%[6,59]。此外,TA患者对堪萨斯分枝杆菌(84% vs. 11%)和禽分枝杆菌(78% vs. 15%)特异性抗原的过敏反应比非TA患者更常见[6]。活动性TA在结核性淋巴结炎患者中更为常见(TA组为21%,肺结核病组为1%)[34]。位于主动脉旁或肠系膜淋巴结与TA炎症血管密切相关的结核性淋巴结炎已被报道[34]。在合并肺外结核的TA患者中,硬结超过10 mm的PPD也更常见(92.5% vs. 89%)[6]。患有和不患有结核病的患者TA

的临床和血管造影特征是无法区分的[34]。TA 的组织病理学特征与结核病变相似,包括肉芽肿性炎症和郎格汉斯型巨细胞[1,24]。在 TA 患者的主动脉组织中发现了与结核分枝杆菌相关的基因序列,包括 IS6110 和 HupB 基因,提示动脉炎与潜伏感染的关系[55]。动脉病变附近淋巴结结节的显示和无半乳糖 IgG 水平的升高也可能代表 TB 和 TA 之间的联系[1]。

另一方面,使用抗 TNF 治疗缓解 TA 患者与分枝杆菌感染的发生无关,这是合理的推断,如果 TA 是由活动性或潜伏性结核感染引起的,抗 TNF 药物应该加重临床反应明显的 TB[6]。Quantiferon-TB Gold Test 通过测量 T 细胞干扰素-γ 体外释放对结核分枝杆菌高度特异的抗原的反应来检测结核病感染,在 TA 和对照组中显示出类似的阳性结果,表明 TA 患者的 TB 感染率并不高于普通人群[24]。未检测到结核(肺源性和肺外源性)与 TA 之间关于 HLA-B 等位基因的任何遗传关系[56]。在合并 TA 和 TB 的患者中,结核不影响 TA 的临床病程[34]。

在 TA 中,以单核细胞(淋巴细胞、巨噬细胞、浆细胞和巨细胞)浸润为特征的炎症始于中外膜交界处的血管周围,累及整个外膜和中层的外 1/3[29,55,58]。Intimae 保持正常,直到它涉及纤维化[55]。可见巨细胞肉芽肿性反应、板层坏死、弹力纤维碎裂和平滑肌细胞丢失[58]。有反应性纤维化、内侧瘢痕形成和血管化[58]。在愈合阶段,纤维化涉及血管的所有三层[58]。包括内膜和外膜纤维化以及中膜退变在内的组织病理学改变导致狭窄或动脉瘤形成[29]。该疾病的病因尚不清楚,但有人认为与遗传、感染或环境因素有关的自身免疫基础相关[58]。TA 与结核病有临床相关性。尽管存在这种关联,但到目前为止还不能证明结核病和 TA 之间的确切联系。

人们普遍认为结核分枝杆菌抗原可以刺激 T 细胞产生针对血管壁的自身免疫反应,从而导致 TA 的发病[6,26,59]。在 TA 患者中发现抗结核杆菌蛋白[包括 65 kDa 热休克蛋白(HSP65)]的抗体滴度显著增加[19,59]。在这种情况下,HSP65 是最常被强调的蛋白质。热休克蛋白广泛存在于从细菌到人类的各种物种中,它们构成了一种古老的细胞内自我防御系统,具有清道夫活性,可以保护细胞蛋白免于变性[1,6,52]。它们表现为细胞压力的结果,包括感染、血压升高、内质网超载、氧化/还原失衡、机械压力和炎症[6,52]。结果表明,人 60 kDa 热休克蛋白(HSP60)与 HSP65 同源,TA 和肺结核患者均具有较高的 HSP60 和 HSP65 抗体 IgG 同型反应率[1,6]。这些抗体可能与导致自身免疫性血管损伤和血管疾病的人类血管自身抗原发生交叉反应[1,6,19,29,34,59]。不仅在 TA 中,HSP65 还与人类的各种风湿性疾病有关[1]。

另一种被提出的机制是无半乳糖 IgG 水平升高,在分枝杆菌疾病和几种自身免疫性疾病,包括类风湿性关节炎、炎症性肠病和 TA[59]中都显著升高。此外,促炎细胞因子,包括白细胞介素-18 和肿瘤坏死因子-α,有助于抗结核感染和肉芽肿形成的免疫作用,可能与 TA 的发病有关,因为在 TA 患者中 IL-18 和 TNF-α 表达上调[59]。虽然结核分枝杆菌从未在活动性或非活动性动脉炎患者的动脉组织中被直接证实[6],但在 TA 患者的主动脉组织中存在结核分枝杆菌 IS6110 和 HupB 基因序列,提示 TB 可能在 TA 中直接诱导炎症反应,而不是一种自身免疫机制[34,55]。此外,对于 TA 的病因,建议接种卡介苗[6,29]。

12.6 动脉粥样硬化

动脉粥样硬化是心血管疾病的主要病理,根据 WHO 的数据,心血管疾病占全球死亡人数的 1/3。虽然没有临床证据表明肺结核患者动脉粥样硬化的发展增加[52],但研究表明,患有 TB 或 EPTB 的患者患急性心肌梗死和不稳定型心绞痛的风险增加 40%,缺血性中风的风险增加 50%[19]。结核与动脉粥样硬化的关系尚不清楚,但应考虑结核病程中的某些机制可能与动脉粥样硬化的发生或发展有关。

很难生长的细胞内生物(巨细胞病毒、单纯疱疹病毒、肺炎衣原体和幽门螺杆菌)与动脉粥样硬化之间存在联系,因为它们的慢性或潜伏感染习惯可能导致持续的炎症,导致动脉粥样硬化斑块的形成[19,52]。动脉粥样硬化主要是一种炎症性疾病。活化的白细胞(包括 T 淋巴细胞和巨噬细胞)和炎症标志物(包括 C 反应蛋白、纤维蛋白原、血清淀粉样蛋白、白细胞介素、肿瘤坏死因子-α 和黏附分子)与动脉粥样硬化的进展有关[52]。结核分枝杆菌病与被指控导致动脉粥样硬化的微生物有相似的特征,并类似地诱导慢性炎症,这可能在动脉粥样硬化中起作用。

热休克蛋白抗体的交叉反应可能与动脉粥样硬化有关,因为内皮细胞在各种应激源激活时会表达热休克蛋白[19,61]。据报道,抗 HSP65 抗体与颈动脉粥样硬化显著相关[19]。动脉粥样硬化患者的热休克蛋白抗体效价较高[52,61]。此外,还发现在动脉粥样硬化斑块中存在对热休克蛋白有特异性反应的 T 细胞[61]。如上所述,针对结核分枝杆菌热休克蛋白 65 产生的抗体可以通过分子模仿诱导 T 和 B 细胞对人热休克蛋白 60 的自身反应,这可能在动脉粥样硬化的发展中起作用[52]。卡介苗免疫动物中的抗 HSP60 效价与动脉粥样硬化斑块的形成相关[52]。

结核诱导自由基的产生,如活性氮中间产物和活性氧物种,这会增强患者的氧化应激并降低抗氧化活性[17,44]。氧化/还原失衡与低密度脂蛋白(low density lipoprotein,LDL)氧化有关,LDL 氧化通过内皮功能障碍、黏附分子表达和泡沫细胞形成在动脉粥样硬化的发病机制中起核心作用。结核病患者的氧化/还原失衡可能与低密度脂蛋白对氧化的易感性增加有关,从而使结核病患者患动脉粥样硬化的风险更高[44]。

12.7 深静脉血栓形成

静脉血栓栓塞(venous thromboembolism,VTE)有几个典型的危险因素,感染被认为是其中之一。此外,结核病也是 VTE 的独立危险因素。在登坦(Dentan)等人的报告中,结核感染过程中发生的炎症、淤积和高凝状态可导致静脉血栓栓塞[25,31]。结合 33 048 852 例住院和门诊资料[11],建立了无潜在凝血障碍的肺结核病与 VTE 的关联。结核病患者中 VTE 的患病率为 2%～4%[11,25]。以优势比(odds ratio,OR)表示的结核患者发生 VTE 的风险接近肿瘤(1.55 vs. 1.62),后者是众所周知的 VTE 危险因素[11]。TB 可由于血小板聚集增加、血小板增多、纤维蛋白原、因子Ⅷ、纤溶酶原激活物抑制物 1 血浆和抗磷脂抗体水平升高以及抗凝血酶Ⅲ和蛋白 C 水平降低而产生高凝状态[11,25,31]。此外,腹膜后淋巴结压迫静脉可能导致瘀血和血栓形成[11,31]。结核杆菌和炎症引起的内皮损伤或利福平的使用可能参与了 VTE 的发病[25]。除了深静脉血栓和肺栓塞外,在肺结核患者中还报告了包括脑静脉窦或肝静脉在内的不寻常部位的血栓形成[25]。

高凝状态在开始抗结核治疗后恢复[31]。结核病患者的 VTE 的治疗应包括抗凝和抗结核治疗[25]。维持标准 INR 水平可能很困难,由于利福平诱导的高凝状态,可能需要高剂量的华法林,因为利福平是一种细胞色素 P450 诱导剂,可以增加抗凝剂的清除[31]。

VTE 是结核病患者的独立预后因素,与死亡率独立相关(OR=3.87)[11]。

同时患有结核病和 VTE 的患者的病死率(15%)高于单独患有结核病的患者(2.7%)和单独患有 VTE 的患者(2.5%)[11]。

参考文献

[1] Aggarwal A, Chag M, Sinha N, Naik S. Takayasu's arteritis: role of Mycobacterium tuberculosis and its 65 kDa heat shock protein. Int J Cardiol. 1996; 55: 49 - 55.

[2] Alkhuja S, Miller A. Tuberculosis and sudden death: a case report and review. Heart Lung J Acute Crit Care. 2001; 30: 388 - 391. https://doi.org/10.1067/mhl.2001.118304.

[3] Allins AD, Wagner WH, Cossman DV, et al. Tuberculous infection of the descending thoracic and abdominal aorta: case report and literature review. Ann Vasc Surg. 1999; 13: 439 - 444. https://doi.org/10.1007/s100169900280.

[4] Amonkar G, Rupani A, Shah V, Parmar H. Sudden death in tuberculous myocarditis. Cardiovasc Pathol. 2009; 18: 247 - 248. https://doi.org/10.1016/j.carpath.2007.12.016.

[5] Biedrzycki OJ, Baithun SI. TB-related sudden death (TBRSD) due to myocarditis complicating miliary TB. Am J Forensic Med Pathol. 2006; 27: 335 - 336. https://doi.org/10.1097/01.paf.0000233633.16185.32.

[6] Castillo-Martínez D, Amezcua-Guerra LM. Self-reactivity against stress-induced cell molecules: the missing link between Takayasu's arteritis and tuberculosis? Med Hypotheses. 2012; 78: 485 - 488. https://doi.org/10.1016/j.mehy.2012.01.012.

[7] Cherian G. Diagnosis of tuberculous aetiology in pericardial effusions. Postgrad Med J. 2004; 80: 262 - 266.

[8] Choudhary SK, Bhan A, Talwar S, et al. Tubercular pseudoaneurysms of aorta. Ann Thorac Surg. 2001; 72: 1239 - 1244.

[9] Cinar B, Enç Y, Göksel O, et al. Chronic constrictive tuberculous pericarditis: risk factors and outcome of pericardiectomy. Int J Tuberc Lung Dis. 2006; 10: 701 - 706.

[10] Clough RE, Topple JA, Zayed HA, et al. Endovascular repair of a tuberculous mycotic thoracic aortic aneurysm with a custom-made device. J Vasc Surg. 2010; 51: 1272 - 1275. https://doi.org/10.1016/j.jvs.2009.12.047.

[11] Dentan C, Epaulard O, Seynaeve D, et al. Active tuberculosis and venous thromboembolism: association according to international classification of diseases, ninth revision hospital discharge diagnosis codes. Clin Infect Dis. 2014; 58: 495 - 501. https://doi.org/10.1093/cid/cit780.

[12] Desai N, Desai S, Chaddha U, Gable B. Tuberculous myopericarditis: a rare presentation in an immunocompetent host. BMJ Case Rep. 2013; 2013: bcr2012007749. https://doi.org/10.1136/bcr - 2012 - 007749.

[13] Díaz-Peromingo JA, Mariño-Callejo AI, González-González C, et al. Tuberculous myocarditis presenting as long QT syndrome. Eur J Intern Med. 2000; 11: 340 - 342.

[14] Dogan S, Memis A, Kale A, Buket S. Endovascular stent graft placement in the treatment of ruptured tuberculous pseudoaneurysm of the descending thoracic aorta: case report and review of the literature. Cardiovasc Intervent Radiol. 2009; 32: 572-576. https://doi.org/10.1007/s00270-008-9456-8.

[15] Golden MP, Vikram HR. Extrapulmonary tuberculosis: an overview. Am Fam Physician. 2005; 72: 1761-1768.

[16] Golzarian J, Cheng J, Giron F, Bilfinger TV. Tuberculous pseudoaneurysm of the descending thoracic aorta: successful treatment by surgical excision and primary repair. Tex Heart Inst J. 1999; 26: 232-235.

[17] Guilford T, Morris D, Gray D, Venketaraman V. Atherosclerosis: pathogenesis and increased occurrence in individuals with HIV and Mycobacterium tuberculosis infection. HIV AIDS (Auckl). 2010; 2: 211-218. https://doi.org/10.2147/HIV.S11977.

[18] Gupta MD, Yadav N, Palleda GM. Granulomatous tubercular myocarditis: a rare cause of heart failure in the young. Cardiol Young. 2013; 23: 740-741. https://doi.org/10.1017/S1047951113000723.

[19] Huaman MA, Henson D, Ticona E, et al. Tuberculosis and cardiovascular disease: linking the epidemics. Trop Dis Travel Med Vaccines. 2015; 1: 10. https://doi.org/10.1186/s40794-015-0014-5.

[20] Ikezawa T, Iwatsuka Y, Naiki K, et al. Tuberculous pseudoaneurysm of the descending thoracic aorta: a case report and literature review of surgically treated cases. J Vasc Surg. 1996; 24: 693-697.

[21] Irdem A, Baspinar O, Kucukosmanoglu E. Dilated cardiomyopathy due to miliary tuberculosis. Anadolu Kardiyol Derg/Anatol J Cardiol. 2013; 13: 499-500. https://doi.org/10.5152/akd.2013.152.

[22] Jain AK, Chauhan RS, Dhammi IK, et al. Tubercular pseudoaneurysm of aorta: a rare association with vertebral tuberculosis. Spine J. 2007; 7: 249-253. https://doi.org/10.1016/j.spinee.2006.04.021.

[23] Kannangara DW, Salem FA, Rao BS, Thadepalli H. Cardiac tuberculosis: TB of the endocardium. Am J Med Sci. 1984; 287: 45-47.

[24] Karadag O, Aksu K, Sahin A, et al. Assessment of latent tuberculosis infection in Takayasu arteritis with tuberculin skin test and Quantiferon-TB Gold test. Rheumatol Int. 2010; 30: 1483-1487. https://doi.org/10.1007/s00296-010-1444-z.

[25] Kechaou I, Cherif E, Ben Hassine L, Khalfallah N. Deep vein thrombosis and tuberculosis: a causative link? BMJ Case Rep. 2014; 2014: bcr2013200807. https://doi.org/10.1136/bcr-2013-200807.

[26] Khemiri M, Douira W, Barsaoui S. Co-occurrence of Takayasu's arteritis and tuberculosis: report of a Tunisian pediatric case. Ann Pediatr Cardiol. 2016; 9: 75-78. https://doi.org/10.4103/0974-2069.171398.

[27] Khurana R, Shalhoub J, Verma A, et al. Tubercular myocarditis presenting with ventricular tachycardia. Nat Clin Pract Cardiovasc Med. 2008; 5: 169-174. https://doi.org/10.1038/ncpcardio1111.

[28] Kolhari VB, Bhairappa S, Prasad NM, Manjunath CN. Tuberculosis: still an enigma. Presenting as mycotic aneurysm of aorta. BMJ Case Rep. 2013; 2013.

https://doi.org/10.1136/bcr-2013-008869.
[29] Kothari SS. Aetiopathogenesis of Takayasu's arteritis and BCG vaccination: the missing link? Med Hypotheses. 1995; 45: 227-230.
[30] Kouchoukos NT, Blackstone EH, Doty DB, et al. Pericardial disease. In: Kirklin/Barrat-Boyes cardiac surgery. 3rd ed. Philadelphia: Churchill Livingstone; 2003. p. 1779-1795.
[31] Kumarihamy K, Ralapanawa D, Jayalath W. A rare complication of pulmonary tuberculosis: a case report. BMC Res Notes. 2015; 8: 39. https://doi.org/10.1186/s13104-015-0990-6.
[32] Li F-P, Wang X-F, Xiao Y-B. Endovascular stent graft placement in the treatment of a ruptured tuberculous pseudoaneurysm of the descending thoracic aorta secondary to Pott's disease of the spine. J Card Surg. 2012; 27: 75-77. https://doi.org/10.1111/j.1540-8191.2011.01343.x.
[33] Li H, Li R, Qu J, et al. Ventricular tachycardia in a disseminated MDR-TB patient: a case report and brief review of literature. Front Med. 2014; 8: 259-263. https://doi.org/10.1007/s11684-014-0321-7.
[34] Lim AY, Lee GY, Jang SY, et al. Comparison of clinical characteristics in patients with Takayasu arteritis with and without concomitant tuberculosis. Heart Vessel. 2016; 31: 1277-1284. https://doi.org/10.1007/s00380-015-0731-8.
[35] Liu A, Hu Y, Coates A. Sudden cardiac death and tuberculosis — How much do we know? Tuberculosis. 2012; 92: 307-313. https://doi.org/10.1016/j.tube.2012.02.002.
[36] Long R, Guzman R, Greenberg H, et al. Tuberculous mycotic aneurysm of the aorta: review of published medical and surgical experience. Chest. 1999; 115: 522-531.
[37] Maisch B, Soler-Soler J, Hatle L, Ristic AD. Pericardial diseases. In: Camm AJ, Lüscher TF, Serruys P, editors. The ESC textbook of cardiovascular medicine. Blackwell Publishing; 2006. p. 517-534. Massachusetts, USA.
[38] Mangi AA, Torchiana DF. Pericardial disease. In: Cohn LH, editor. Cardiac surgery in the adult. 3rd ed. New York: McGraw-Hill; 2008. p. 1465-1478.
[39] Manika K, Efthymiou C, Damianidis G, et al. Miliary tuberculosis in a patient with tuberculous mycotic aneurysm of the abdominal aorta: case report and review of the literature. Respir Med Case Rep. 2017; 21: 30-35. https://doi.org/10.1016/j.rmcr.2017.03.010.
[40] Mayosi BM, Burgess LJ, Doubell AF. Tuberculous pericarditis. Circulation. 2005; 112: 3608-3616. https://doi.org/10.1161/CIRCULATIONAHA.105.543066.
[41] Michira BN, Alkizim FO, Matheka DM. Patterns and clinical manifestations of tuberculous myocarditis: a systematic review of cases. Pan Afr Med J. 2015; 21: 118. https://doi.org/10.11604/pamj.2015.21.118.4282.
[42] Mohan A, Thachil A, Sundar G, et al. Ventricular tachycardia and tuberculous lymphadenopathy: Sign of myocardial tuberculosis? J Am Coll Cardiol. 2015; 65: 218-220.
[43] Mutyaba AK, Ntsekhe M. Tuberculosis and the heart. Cardiol Clin. 2017; 35: 135-144. https://doi.org/10.1016/j.ccl.2016.08.007.
[44] Nezami N, Ghorbanihaghjo A, Rashtchizadeh N, et al. Atherogenic changes of

low-density lipoprotein susceptibility to oxidation, and antioxidant enzymes in pulmonary tuberculosis. Atherosclerosis. 2011; 217: 268-273. https://doi.org/10.1016/j.atherosclerosis.2011.03.025.

[45] Ntsekhe M, Wiysonge CS, Commerford PJ, Mayosi BM. The prevalence and outcome of effusive constrictive pericarditis: a systematic review of the literature. Cardiovasc J Afr. 2012; 23: 281-285. https://doi.org/10.5830/CVJA-2011-072.

[46] Ohtsuka T, Kotsuka Y, Yagyu K, et al. Tuberculous pseudoaneurysm of the thoracic aorta. Ann Thorac Surg. 1996; 62: 1831-1834.

[47] Palaniswamy C, Kumar U, Selvaraj DR, et al. Tuberculous mycotic aneurysm of aortic root: an unusual cause of cardiac tamponade. Trop Dr. 2009; 39: 112-113. https://doi.org/10.1258/td.2008.080199.

[48] Parkhurst GF, Dekcer JP. Bacterial aortitis and mycotic aneurysm of the aorta: a report of twelve cases. Am J Pathol. 1955; 31: 821-835.

[49] Pathirana U, Kularatne S, Karunaratne S, et al. Ascending aortic aneurysm caused by Mycobacterium tuberculosis. BMC Res Notes. 2015; 8: 659. https://doi.org/10.1186/s13104-015-1667-x.

[50] Rajesh S, Sricharan KN, Jayaprakash K, Monteiro FNP. Cardiac involvement in patients with pulmonary tuberculosis. J Clin Diagn Res. 2011; 5: 440-442.

[51] Reuter H, Burgess L, van Vuuren W, Doubell A. Diagnosing tuberculous pericarditis. QJM. 2006; 99: 827-839. https://doi.org/10.1093/qjmed/hcl123.

[52] Rota S, Rota S. Mycobacterium tuberculosis complex in atherosclerosis. Acta Med Okayama. 2005; 59: 247-251.

[53] Roubille F, Gahide G, Granier M, et al. Likely tuberculous myocarditis mimicking an acute coronary syndrome. Intern Med. 2008; 47: 1699-1701.

[54] Silingardi E, Rivasi F, Santunione AL, Garagnani L. Sudden death from tubercular myocarditis. J Forensic Sci. 2006; 51: 667-669. https://doi.org/10.1111/j.1556-4029.2006.00117.x.

[55] Soto ME, Del Carmen Ávila-Casado M, Huesca-Gómez C, et al. Detection of IS6110 and HupB gene sequences of Mycobacterium tuberculosis and bovisin the aortic tissue of patients with Takayasu's arteritis. BMC Infect Dis. 2012; 12: 194. https://doi.org/10.1186/1471-2334-12-194.

[56] Soto ME, Vargas-Alarcón G, Cicero-Sabido R, et al. Comparison distribution of HLA-B alleles in Mexican patients with Takayasu arteritis and tuberculosis. Hum Immunol. 2007; 68: 449-453. https://doi.org/10.1016/j.humimm.2007.01.004.

[57] Trautner BW, Darouiche RO. Tuberculous pericarditis: optimal diagnosis and management. Clin Infect Dis. 2001; 33: 954-961. https://doi.org/10.1086/322621.

[58] Vaideeswar P, Deshpande JR. Pathology of Takayasu arteritis: a brief review. Ann Pediatr Cardiol. 2013; 6: 52-58. https://doi.org/10.4103/0974-2069.107235.

[59] Walters HM, Aguiar CL, MacDermott EJ, et al. Takayasu arteritis presenting in the context of active tuberculosis. J Clin Rheumatol. 2013; 19: 344-347. https://doi.org/10.1097/RHU.0b013e31829ce750.

[60] Zhang C, Chen B, Gu Y, et al. Tuberculous abdominal aortic pseudoaneurysm

with renal and vertebral tuberculosis: a case and literature review. J Infect Dev Ctries. 2014; 8: 1216-1221.
[61] Zhang Y, Xiong Q, Hu X, et al. A novel atherogenic epitope from Mycobacterium tuberculosis heat shock protein 65 enhances atherosclerosis in rabbit and LDL receptor-deficient mice. Heart Vessel. 2012; 27: 411-418. https://doi.org/10.1007/s00380-011-0183-8.

13
皮肤结核

萨马拉·A.密目和齐亚德·A.密目

结核病,一种由结核分枝杆菌引起的感染性疾病,已经存在了几千年,直到今天它仍是影响全球的公共卫生健康问题。据世界卫生组织统计,全球约有20%~40%的人口受结核影响,仅在2015年就有1040万新发结核病病例(包括120万HIV阳性患者),其中男性590万例,女性350万例,儿童100万例。总体而言,90%的病例为成人,10%为儿童,男女比例为1.6∶1。全球大部分的结核以肺结核为主,但是这种细菌可以以肺外结核的形式影响身体其他任何器官,包括皮肤(约8.4%~13.7%)。这使得皮肤结核成为一种相对少见的传染病,仅占肺外结核病例的1%~2%,约占所有皮肤疾病的0.1%~1%。只有5%~10%的结核分枝杆菌感染会导致结核病的发生,体现了MTB的低毒力。皮肤结核随着合并HIV感染、耐多药结核病的增加以及近年来生物制剂特别是抗肿瘤坏死因子(Anti-TNF)治疗应用的增加而增加[2]。

13.1 分类

临床表现主要取决于感染途径、细胞免疫和结核杆菌毒性。各种局部因素也起作用,如皮肤屏障受损、血管形成、淋巴管引流以及邻近区域淋巴结[3]。根据感染方式和宿主的免疫状态,有多种表现形式和形态分类。皮肤结核分为三大类:

  1. 外源性感染
  2. 内源性感染
  3. 血行播散

13.1.1 外源性感染

结核性下疳是在没有接触或免疫结核分枝杆菌的情况下,通过接种MTB到患者的皮肤或黏膜中而造成的损害。细菌进入皮肤可能是由于皮肤或黏膜损伤导致的皮肤屏障受损,如伤口、文身、穿孔、拔牙、仪式性割礼和人工呼吸[4],常见于儿童的面部和四肢。结核性下疳表现为无痛不愈合的丘疹或溃疡,可达到 5 cm[5],通常发生于接种后 2~4 周。溃疡浅,边缘破坏,基底呈颗粒状或出血性,在 3~8 周内发展至局部淋巴结。在数周至数月后可能形成冷脓肿,可能穿孔导致窦道形成。若不治疗,病变可持续一年,最终愈合留下瘢痕。50%的病例局部淋巴结缓慢消退且可能钙化[5]。

如果免疫功能受损,可能发生疾病的复发或血行播散。

黏膜病变可表现为结膜水肿或溃疡伴局部淋巴结炎[6]。口腔病变虽然罕见,但也有报道[7]。

早期病变的组织病理学表现为混合性真皮炎性浸润和大量抗酸杆菌。3~6 周后,病灶和区域淋巴结内会形成结核样肉芽肿,同时可能伴有干酪性坏死[8]。

疣状皮肤结核(疣状肺结核)发生在再次接触结核杆菌或接种疫苗后具有中到高免疫力的个体。多发生于成人手部或儿童下肢。开始常呈现为带有淡紫色环的伴有疼痛的孤立性硬丘疹,随后缓慢发展成无症状的过度角化的疣状斑块,边缘不规则延伸呈现出锯齿状外观[9]。如果不治疗,病变会缓慢生长,持续多年。偶尔会自行愈合,留下萎缩瘢痕。

这类病变的组织病理学表现为明显的过度角化和假上皮瘤样增生,并伴有真皮干酪性肉芽肿。如果仔细检查标本,可找到抗酸杆菌[5,8]。

13.1.2 内源性感染

皮肤感染是皮下组织、淋巴结、泪腺或导管、骨骼和关节等感染病灶直接蔓延引起的。

据报道,皮肤瘰疬是 10 岁以下儿童最常见的皮肤结核[10]。在感染病灶上,有一红蓝色、质硬、活动可的无症状结节。随后可能在数月时间内液化、破裂,形成溃疡和窦道。溃疡可呈线形或锯齿状,边缘呈蓝色,底部有肉芽组织[9]。瘢痕和肉芽组织可能导致不规则的蕈状瘤。

病理组织学显示病灶中心有干酪坏死，周围有结核性肉芽肿。坏死的皮肤碎片中常可分离出抗酸杆菌。

腔口结核（皮肤开口结核）在肺部、肠道、生殖器或泌尿系统的晚期感染患者中，大量活结核杆菌经天然开口接种到附近的黏膜或皮肤而形成。这些患者病情严重，免疫力低下。病变通常发生在口腔黏膜，呈红色疼痛性结节，迅速形成浅溃疡，边缘呈蓝色，无法愈合[9]。

13.1.3 血行播散型结核

通过血行播散或淋巴结播散感染皮肤称为血行播散型结核。寻常性狼疮是最常见的血行传播形式，发生在具有中高度免疫力的个体中[4]。它也可能是接种疫苗、接种卡介苗、直接扩散或淋巴传播而引起。超过80%的病变位于头部和颈部，尤其是鼻子周围[9]。最初表现为红棕色斑块，在散斑显微镜上有典型的苹果果冻外观。随后病变逐渐增大，变硬，隆起，呈褐色。有5种主要的临床表现。斑块是最常见的表现，为红棕色，表面光滑或呈银屑病样，边缘不规则，过度角化。这些病变均有不同程度的瘢痕形成。溃疡或致残类型是破坏性的，侵入深部组织和软骨，留下坏死的结痂和瘢痕。增生型病变的特征是溃疡和坏死，但瘢痕很小，当鼻或耳软骨受到侵犯时容易造成毁容。肿瘤样病变，光滑或过度角化，通常累及耳垂，可引起淋巴水肿和血管扩张。暂时性免疫抑制后，常表现为丘疹结节。

皮肤活检显示真皮上部和中部周边有伴淋巴细胞的结核样肉芽肿，病变偶尔会出现在中央。病变为少菌性病变，但部分切片可见抗酸杆菌[8]。

结核性牙龈瘤又称转移性结核性脓肿，是一种罕见的血液播散形式，在宿主免疫力低下，可导致单一或多个皮肤或皮下病变。脓肿通常是非压痛性的，可以表现为一个波动性脓肿结节或坚实的皮下结节[9]。上覆的皮肤最终会破裂，导致溃疡和窦道。结核菌可以从分泌物中分离出来[5,9]。

急性粟粒型结核：又称播散性结核，是一种罕见的危及生命的疾病，通常影响儿童和免疫低下患者。最初出现多发性蓝褐色丘疹、水泡和出血性病变。随后水泡坏死和溃烂。组织病理学显示真皮内有慢性非特异性炎症浸润，周围有坏死和脓肿形成，并伴有大量抗酸杆菌。

1896年，达利尔首次描述了结核疹，它是由于高免疫力个体对结核菌或其产物过敏所致。他们的特点是结核菌素试验呈阳性,对抗结核治疗有阳性反应,并且很难从机体中分离出来。

真正的结核疹可分为三大类:

1. 小丘疹: 瘰疬性苔藓
2. 丘疹: 丘疹坏死性结核
3. 结节性: Bazin 硬红斑,结节性结核疹

瘰疬性苔藓是一种少见的苔藓样疹,多见于儿童及青年人。躯干和四肢近端通常出现一批无症状的肤色、淡黄色或红棕色的苔藓样丘疹。受累皮肤的组织病理学表现为小叶周围非干酪性结核样肉芽肿,不易找到结核杆菌[8]。

丘疹坏死性结核主要表现为青壮年四肢的暗红色坏死丘疹。病变愈合时会形成一块斑片状的瘢痕。病变的组织病理学表现为表皮溃烂,真皮厚度不一,有坏死区。病变周围环绕一层组织细胞,邻近血管可见血管炎、纤维素样坏死或血栓形成。

Bazin 硬红斑的病变局限于皮下脂肪,通常位于小腿后部。病变可溃烂并产生浅溃疡,边缘不规则呈蓝色,是一种伴有中性粒细胞血管炎的小叶性脂膜炎。

13.2 非结核分枝杆菌

非结核分枝杆菌感染,如以前所命名的,主要发生在免疫功能低下的宿主中。在免疫功能正常的宿主中,感染穿透皮肤后,通常是局限性的,而在免疫功能低下的患者中有传播的趋势。这一类分枝杆菌有很多种,但引起皮肤病的最常见的是偶然分枝杆菌复合体(偶然分枝杆菌、龟分枝杆菌和脓肿分枝杆菌)、海洋分枝杆菌、嗜血分枝杆菌和溃烂分枝杆菌。这些生物广泛分布于环境中,可以在土壤、水、植物、皮肤共生生物和一些动物中找到[4,5]。

偶然分枝杆菌复合体是一种快速生长的分枝杆菌,能够同时在免疫正常和免疫受损的宿主中引起疾病。前者有外伤导致局部损伤的病史,后者则是无穿透性损伤史的播散性疾病。局部疾病可能表现为结节、脓肿、溃疡、蜂窝组织炎和窦道。播散性皮肤病表现为多个结节,无特殊类型。

鱼缸肉芽肿或游泳池肉芽肿是由接种海洋真菌引起的皮肤病。它是从

盐水和淡水中分离出来的。潜伏期最早为 2~3 周,最晚可达 9 个月。病变开始是结节或脓疱,后来可能形成溃疡或脓肿,最终形成疣状斑块。病变通常是多发性的,可沿淋巴管引流呈孢子丝状扩张。

布鲁里溃疡首次出现在 1897 年,乌干达当地用来描述溃烂分枝杆菌引起的皮肤病[9]。据报道,该病主要发生在热带和亚热带河流地区。传播方式尚不清楚。大多数患者是 15 岁以下的儿童。他们表现为一个质硬可活动的皮下结节,可发展成无痛性浅表坏死性溃疡,坏死边缘受损。溃疡通常是单一的,但会在数周内长到几厘米大小。

嗜血分枝杆菌的自然栖息地和传播方式尚不清楚。它影响免疫功能低下的患者,尤其是器官移植和长期使用免疫抑制剂的患者。患者四肢有多个疼痛的紫罗兰色结节,可发展为溃疡或脓肿。皮肤病可能伴随着全身症状,如体重减轻、腱鞘炎、骨髓炎、关节积液或呼吸道症状[9]。

13.3　治疗

目前对皮肤结核的治疗选择仅限于常规的抗结核药物,以及在某些适应证下的一些外科干预措施(手术切除病变和矫正畸形)。使用的标准治疗药物包括异烟肼、利福平、吡嗪酰胺、乙胺丁醇和链霉素。值得注意的是,大多数报告的皮肤结核病例对常用药物敏感,耐药皮肤结核非常罕见。皮肤结核的治疗类似于肺结核,分两个阶段使用联合抗结核药物:强化或杀菌期使用异烟肼、利福平、乙胺丁醇和吡嗪酰胺联合使用 8 周,维持期或灭菌期使用异烟肼和利福平 16 周。在 HIV 阳性的皮肤结核病患者中,治疗的维持期从 16 周延长到 28 周。如果皮肤结核病灶接近自然开口,可使用 2% 乳酸和局部麻醉药。

对于非结核分枝杆菌的皮肤感染,抗结核药物的疗效较差,因此可以根据药敏情况使用多种抗生素来治疗此类感染。这种情况下的治疗通常比较困难,需要较长的疗程。到目前为止,还没有可用于治疗皮肤结核的局部抗结核药物[4]。

参考文献

[1]　Spelta K, Diniz LM. Cutaneous tuberculosis: a 26-year retrospective STUDY in

an endemic area of tuberculosis, Vitória, Espírito Santo, Brazil. Rev Inst Med Trop Sao Paulo. 2016; 58: 49.
[2] Hernandez C, et al. Tuberculosis in the age of biologic therapy. JAAD. 2008; 59 (3): 363-380.
[3] Handog EB, Gabriel TG, Pineda RT. Management of cutaneous tuberculosis. Dermatol Ther. 2008; 21: 154-161.
[4] van Zyl L, du Plessis J, Viljoen J. Cutaneous tuberculosis overview and current treatment regimens. Tuberculosis. 2015; 95: 629-638.
[5] Tappeiner G, Wolf K. Tuberculosis and other mycobacterial infections. Fitz; 1999.
[6] Kakakhel KU, Mohammad S. Tuberculosis of the conjunctiva, eyelid and periocular skin. Pak J Ophthalmol. 1988; 4: 37-40.
[7] Heilman KM, Muschenheim C. Primary cutaneous tuberculosis resulting from mouth-to-mouth respiration. N Engl J Med. 1965; 273: 1035-1036.
[8] Weedon D. Skin pathology. London, United Kingdom: Elsevier Science Limited, 2002.
[9] Bolognia J, Jopizzo J, Rapini R. Dermatology. Spain: Elsevier Limited, 2003.
[10] Sethuraman G, Ramesh V. Cutaneous tuberculosis in children. Pediatr Dermatol. 2013; 30(1): 7-16.

14
眼结核

阿尔祖·塔斯基兰·科梅兹

肺结核是一种由抗酸杆菌结核分枝杆菌引起的呼吸道传染病,最常见累及肺部。它也可以影响身体的任何其他部位,仍然是世界范围内最常见的致病和死亡的原因[1]。

由结核分枝杆菌或牛分枝杆菌、非洲分枝杆菌和微小分枝杆菌引起的眼周或眼内感染被定义为"眼结核"(眼部结核)[2]。

原发眼结核是指无全身受累的眼部结核,或分枝杆菌经眼部侵入人体而发病的结核,继发性眼结核是由远处器官的血行播散或邻近组织(如鼻窦或颅腔)的直接侵入所致的眼部受累。

虽然据估计1.4%的肺结核患者最终会发展为眼结核,但无临床证据表明眼结核与肺结核有关[3]。此外,近60%有肺外结核感染的患者可能并没有肺结核感染的证据[1]。

眼结核最常见的临床表现是葡萄膜炎,其中后葡萄膜炎最常见,其次是前葡萄膜炎、全葡萄膜炎和中间葡萄膜炎[4]。

在19世纪,结核病被认为是葡萄膜炎的常见病因。在20世纪40年代,盖顿(Guyton)和伍兹(Woods)认为肺结核是80%的肉芽肿性葡萄膜炎的病因[5]。然而,随着新的诊断试验,眼结核的诊断标准变得更加严格,以前未确定病因的结节病、弓形虫病和组织胞浆菌病得到了界定;结核分枝杆菌引起的葡萄膜炎病例数随之下降[5]。自20世纪80年代以来,文献报道中提到仅有0~4%葡萄膜炎的病因是结核病[5-9]。据报道,眼结核的特定地区患病率在印度为0.4%~9.8%,在中国为4%,在日本为7%[10-13]。

据报道,结核病在丹麦是慢性虹膜睫状体炎、播散性脉络膜炎和外周炎的主要病因,在俄罗斯是后葡萄膜炎的主要病因[14,15]。

辛格(Singh)等人在他们的眼内液PCR研究中报道30%的葡萄膜炎患

者有感染源，2/3是眼内结核[12]。

在土耳其的三级中心，结核病被认为是0.3%的葡萄膜炎患者的病因[16]。

14.1 体征和症状

视力减退、畏光和眼睛发红是最常见的症状。然而，患者也可能没有症状或有头痛、闪光和飞蚊症等主诉。

14.2 眼结核的临床表现

眼结核是肺结核和肺外结核血源性播散造成的，经结膜原发性眼部感染在儿童中很少见。症状性疾病通常是由于眼部组织中静止性病变的重新激活，而不是原发感染。

肺结核分枝杆菌抗原超敏反应引起的眼部病变是眼结核的另一种形式[1]。

眼结核通常是单侧不对称的。可能影响眼表、眼睑、结膜、角膜、巩膜、葡萄膜、脉络膜、视网膜、眼眶、泪腺和延伸至中枢神经系统的视神经[5,17]。

14.3 主要临床表现

1. 葡萄膜炎

是眼结核最突出的临床表现，主要表现为后葡萄膜炎，其次是前葡萄膜炎、全葡萄膜炎和中间葡萄膜炎。眼结核有各种各样的葡萄膜炎表现，因此葡萄膜炎成为是结核病的一个重要伪装。

后葡萄膜炎合并播散性脉络膜炎是结核性葡萄膜炎最常见的表现，通常是双侧的[18]。单侧或双侧后极可见直径大小不等的多发、离散的黄色病变（脉络膜结核球）。随着病变的发展，它们的边界可能会变得更加清晰，中心变得更加苍白，从而导致萎缩性瘢痕。随后可能发展为视网膜下新生血管、视网膜下脓肿和脉络膜炎。

急性或慢性肉芽肿性前葡萄膜炎可见羊脂性角化沉淀物、虹膜或房角肉芽肿、后粘连、疱疹、继发性白内障、玻璃体炎和继发性青光眼[19]。中间葡萄膜炎伴有部分扁平炎症状,如雪堆、轻度慢性玻璃体炎、外周血管鞘和外周视网膜脉络膜肉芽肿[19]。

可出现椎间盘水肿、静脉周围炎、血管炎和玻璃炎。

2. 视网膜炎与视网膜血管炎

视网膜表现通常是由于脉络膜表现所致。视网膜血管炎主要发生在视网膜静脉,血管周围有袖带;很少与动脉相关。

3. 视神经病变与神经性视网膜炎

视神经病变可能是微生物直接侵入或对微生物过敏所致。也可能有视神经炎、视盘炎、视盘水肿、球后神经炎和神经视网膜炎等其他表现[19-22]。

4. 眼内炎和全眼炎

这种形式是急性的和进行性的,导致眼前房积脓填充前房和玻璃体腔。视网膜下脓肿可能发生,液化坏死可能导致眼球穿孔[19]。

5. 脉络膜结节

是眼内结核最常见的病变,是分枝杆菌血行传播的指标。

脉络膜结节是一种单侧、淡黄色的病变,边界不清,中心隆起,直径从1~4个视盘大小不等,数量通常少于5个,随着时间的推移,可能会出现色素沉着。黄斑附近或黄斑处的结节会伴有视力减退,其他则无症状。

在一系列尸检中,近50%的病例发现脉络膜结节[23]。

6. 眼眶受累

最常见于儿童,很少有成人病例报告。可发现包括引流的窦道,或放射学证据显示骨质破坏。

7. 结核性结膜炎

通常是单侧的慢性结膜炎,偶尔伴有溃疡、结膜下结节、带蒂息肉、结膜肿块或溃疡。大多数患者没有结核病的全身性表现,提示可能是原发眼结核。

8. 眼睑受累

肺结核也可以表现为眼睑脓肿或结石样肿块。脓肿自发引流可形成引流性窦道。

9. 泪腺受累(泪囊炎)

临床上可能无法与细菌感染区分开来。

10. 巩膜炎

巩膜受累,虽罕见,但也会发生。活检证实存在巩膜炎病例。

11. 扁平苔藓

是一种Ⅳ型超敏反应，表现为角膜上的炎性肿块，可与金黄色葡萄球菌和结核病有关。

12. 伊莱斯病

这是一种罕见的疾病，与结核分枝杆菌无关，但与结核菌素皮肤试验呈阳性有关。它的特点是年轻男性反复发生玻璃体积血。

14.4 诊断

由于疾病的伪装特性，眼结核的诊断常比较困难，并且不可能通过活检来培养和直接观察病原体提供眼结核的确诊依据[24]。可以通过涂片检查和抗酸杆菌染色、眼内组织/液体培养来确诊结核分枝杆菌感染。历史上，证明眼结核的唯一方法是摘除眼球进行组织病理学评估。最近通过玻璃体切割术或脉络膜视网膜活检获得眼内标本，可以在保持眼睛完整的同时获得组织病理学诊断。然而，通常从眼内液中获得的细菌数量较少，难以通过直接镜检和培养试验进行诊断，但干酪化、坏死或眼内炎的病变涂片可发现抗酸染色阳性杆菌[19]。由于眼内液体量的限制，PCR成为一种重要的诊断工具，只需少量标本即可检测。前房积液、玻璃体、视网膜下积液，以及极少数通过玻璃体切除获得的脉络膜视网膜活检标本或视网膜前膜，都可以PCR进行分析[19]。

当无法通过手术获得标本时，评估胸部X线片是否有浸润、空洞或胸腔积液极为重要。可对尿液、脑脊液或痰液进行抗酸染色和培养。

14.5 眼结核诊断标准

虽然目前还没有明确的诊断标准，但在一些文献中报道的眼结核病的诊断标准是：是否存在任何有提示意义的眼部表现，如葡萄膜炎（前、中、后或全葡萄膜炎）、视网膜炎、视网膜血管炎、神经性视网膜炎、视神经病变、眼内炎或全眼炎，与结核患者有接触史，排除任何其他原因引起的葡萄膜炎，皮肤试验阳性，胸片上有陈旧或活动性病变，眼液抗酸杆菌染色或培养证明有结核分枝杆菌，PCR检测提示眼液中有IS6110或其他结核分枝杆菌基因组保守序列，γ-干扰素释放试验（IGRAs）阳性，4~6周内常规抗结核治疗呈阳性反应而无复发[1,25-28]。

这些指南将眼结核分为确诊和临床诊断两类[27-30]。

2015年,古普塔(Gupta)等人提出了新的诊断指南,分为3种类型:确诊、极可能和可能的眼结核[28]。这一新提出的眼结核分类提供了更明确的诊断和更多的病例定义标准[28]。

对四联抗结核药物(异烟肼、利福平、乙胺丁醇、吡嗪酰胺)治疗4~6周有效称为诊断性治疗实验阳性。该疗法应由结核病专家指导,眼科医师应对该疗法的眼部反应进行评估[19,27-30]。

14.6　眼内结核的眼部成像技术

眼底荧光血管造影术是最常见的成像方式,吲哚菁绿血管造影术、光相干体层摄影术(optical coherence tomopraphy,OCT)、眼眶超声和超声生物显微镜术也是常见的成像方式[19,28-29]。

14.7　药物治疗

目前眼结核的治疗包括长期服用四联药物(异烟肼、利福平、乙胺丁醇和吡嗪酰胺)(共9~15个月)[29,30]。

应首选联合治疗,防止产生耐药。CDC建议使用四联药物(异烟肼、利福平、乙胺丁醇和吡嗪酰胺)治疗2个月,然后用两联药物(异烟肼、利福平)治疗4个月。免疫抑制患者的两联药物治疗可延长至7个月[19,31,32]。

目前还不清楚最佳疗程,但建议延长治疗时间[19,32]。

可在4~6周的四联抗结核药物治疗中加用皮质类固醇,以减轻Ⅳ型超敏反应所致的眼部损害。不可单独使用皮质类固醇,以防止潜伏感的再次激活或全身感染的发作[30]。

14.8　抗结核药物的眼部不良反应

乙胺丁醇可能导致剂量相关毒性。所有患者在接受乙胺丁醇治疗前应进行视力、视野检查和色觉检查。剂量低于15 mg/d很少导致眼部不良反应。最常见的毒性体征是视神经病变、获得性红绿色色差、中央暗点、椎间盘水肿、椎间盘充血、乳头周围碎片出血、视神经萎缩、视网膜水肿和黄斑色素改变。接受乙胺丁醇治疗的患者应每2～4周由眼科医师随访一次,剂量超过15 mg/d的患者应每3～6个月随访一次[19,33]。

异烟肼引起视神经炎和视神经萎缩病例报道较少[19]。

眼结核是一种临床表现各异的具有伪装性的疾病,没有检验金标准来确诊。一种经验性诊断方法,包括对临床症状、眼部和全身检查结果的评估,以及通过直接显微镜观测、培养或PCR方法检测到眼内液体和组织中的抗酸杆菌,做出明确诊断后可使用四联药物进行长期抗结核治疗。

参考文献

[1] Shakarchi FI. Ocular tuberculosis: current perspectives. Clin Ophthalmol. 2015; 9: 2223 - 7. https://doi.org/10.2147/OPTH.S65254.

[2] Jabbar A, Khan J, Ullah A, Rehman H, Ali I. Detection of Mycobacterium tuberculosis and Mycobacterium bovis from human sputum samples through multiplex PCR. Pak J Pharm Sci. 2015; 28(4): 1275 - 1280.

[3] Biswas J, Badrinath SS. Ocular morbidity in patients with active systemic tuberculosis. Int Ophthalmol. 1995 - 1996; 19: 293 - 298.

[4] Abu El-Asrar AM, Abouammoh M, Al-Mezaine HS. Tuberculous uveitis. Middle East Afr J Ophthalmol. 2009; 16(4): 188 - 201. https://doi.org/10.4103/0974 - 9233.58421.

[5] Woods AC. Modern concepts of the etiology of uveitis. Am J Ophthalmol. 1960; 50: 1170 - 1187.

[6] Samson MC, Foster CS. Tuberculosis. In: Foster CS, Vitale AT, editors. Diagnosis and treatment of uveitis. Philadelphia: WB Saunders Company; 2002. p. 264 - 272.

[7] Woods AC, Abrahams IW. Uveitis survey sponsored by the American Academy of Ophthalmology and Otolaryngology. Am J Ophthalmol. 1961; 51: 761 - 780.

[8] Henderly DE, Genstler AJ, Smith RE, Rao NA. Changing patterns of uveitis. Am J Ophthalmol. 1987; 103: 131 - 136.

[9] Donahue HC. Ophthalmologic experience in a tuberculosis sanatorium. Am J Ophthalmol. 1967; 64: 742 - 748.

[10] Rathinam SR, Namperumalsamy P. Global variation and pattern changes in epidemiology of uveitis. Indian J Ophthalmol. 2007; 55: 173 - 183.

[11] Yang P, Zhang Z, Zhou H, Li B, Huang X, Gao Y, et al. Clinical patterns and characteristics of uveitis in a tertiary canter for uveitis in China. Curr Eye Res. 2005; 30: 943 - 948.

[12] Singh R, Gupta V, Gupta A. Pattern of uveitis in a referral eye clinic in north India. Indian J Ophthalmol. 2004; 52: 121 - 125.

[13] Wakabayashi T, Morimura Y, Miyamoto Y, Okada AA. Changing pattern of

intraocular inflammatory disease in Japan. Ocul Immunol Inflamm. 2003; 11: 277-286.
[14] Norn M. [Ophthalmic tuberculosis, especially in Denmark]. Dan Medicinhist Arbog. 2001; 212-218.
[15] Khokkanen VM, Iagafarova RK. Clinical and epidemiological characteristics of patients with eye tuberculosisProbl Tuberk. 1998; 6: 14-15.
[16] Kazokoglu H, Onal S, Tugal-Tutkun I, et al. Demographic and clinical features of uveitis in tertiary centers in Turkey. Ophthalmic Epidemiol. 2008; 15: 285-293.
[17] Alvarez S, McCabe WR. Extrapulmonary tuberculosis revisited: a review of experience at Boston City and other hospitals. Medicine (Baltimore). 1984; 63(1): 25-55.
[18] Al-Shakarchi F. Mode of presentations and management of presumed tuberculous uveitis at a referral center. Iraqi Postgrad Med J. 2015; 14(1): 91-95.
[19] Gupta V, Gupta A, Rao NA. Intraocular tuberculosis-an update. Surv Ophthalmol. 2007; 52: 561-587.
[20] Helm CJ, Holland GN. Ocular tuberculosis. Surv Ophthalmol. 1993; 38: 229-256.
[21] Bodaghi B, LeHoang P. Ocular tuberculosis. Curr Opin Ophthalmol. 2000; 11: 443-448.
[22] Ray S, Gragoudas E. Neuroretinitis. Int Ophthalmol Clin. 2001; 41: 83-102.
[23] Slavin RE, Walsh TJ, Pollack AD. Late generalized tuberculosis: a clinical pathologic analysis and comparison of 100 cases in the preantibiotic and antibiotic eras. Medicine (Baltimore). 1980; 59: 352-366.
[24] Varma D, Anand S, Reddy AR, et al. Tuberculosis: an under-diagnosed aetiological agent in uveitis with an effective treatment. Eye (Lond). 2006; 20: 1068-1073.
[25] Feng Y, Diao N, Shao L, et al. Interferon-gamma release assay performance in pulmonary and extrapulmonary tuberculosis. Chabalgoity JA, ed. PLoS One. 2012; 7(3): e32652. https://doi.org/10.1371/journal.pone.0032652.
[26] Ang M, Wong W, Ngan CC, Chee SP. Interferon-gamma release assay as a diagnostic test for tuberculosis-associated uveitis. Eye. 2012; 26(5): 658-665.
[27] Gupta A, Gupta V. Tubercular posterior uveitis. Int Ophthalmol Clin. 2005; 45: 71-88.
[28] Gupta A, Sharma A, Bansal R, Sharma K. Classification of intraocular tuberculosis. Ocul Immunol Inflamm. 2015; 23(1): 7-13. https://doi.org/10.3109/09273948.2014.967358.
[29] Onal S, Tutkun IT. Ocular tuberculosis I: epidemiology, pathogenesis and clinical features. Turk J Ophthalmol. 2011; 41: 171-181.
[30] Onal S, Tutkun IT. Ocular tuberculosis II: diagnosis and treatment. Turk J Ophthalmol. 2011; 41: 182-190.
[31] Bansal R, Gupta A, Gupta V, Dogra MR, Bambery P, Arora SK. Role of antitubercular therapy in uveitis with latent/manifest tuberculosis. Am J Ophthalmol. 2008; 146: 772-779.

[32] Centers for Disease Control and Prevention (CDC); American Thoracic Society. Update: adverse event data and revised American Thoracic Society/CDC recommendations against the use of rifampin and pyrazinamide for treatment of latent tuberculosis infection — United States, 2003. MMWR Morb Mortal Wkly Rep. 2003; 52: 735-739.

[33] Bıçakcı F, Ozeren A, Yerdelen D, Sarica Y. Etambutol kullanımına bağlı optik nöropati. Turkiye Klinikleri J Med Sci. 2005; 25: 460-462.

15
肺外结核的感染控制

露尔·拉卡和格伊尔·穆里奇-奥斯马尼

15.1 简介：结核病的传播

结核病仍然是全球主要的公共卫生问题之一。2015年，估计有1 040万人患上结核病，180万人死于该病，其中40万人合并HIV感染[1,2]。

结核分枝杆菌通过空气传播途径在人与人之间传播，感染者说话、咳嗽或打喷嚏。这些活动产生液体粒子称为液滴核，其中就含有结核分枝杆菌。下列医疗过程中也可能产生这种液滴：痰诱导、支气管镜检查、气管插管、结核性脓肿引流和尸检[3,4]。

1~5 μm的液滴核是传播感染的最高风险。它们在空气中停留较长的时间，并寻找机会进入肺泡腔。这些飞沫只需要携带一种活的结核分枝杆菌就可以传播感染[5]。

结核病的传播受患者的传染性、环境和暴露时间的影响。结核患者的传染性直接取决于携带结核分枝杆菌的液滴核的数量。此外，结核的感染还受其他一些因素的影响：发病地点、咳嗽和痰涂片结果、空洞病变、治疗持续时间以及患者在咳嗽时是否捂住口鼻。

虽然空气传播途径是结核分枝杆菌医疗相关传播的最重要途径，但偶尔也会通过其他途径感染，如支气管镜、器官移植、尸检和给实验动物注射结核分枝杆菌等。

15.2 感染控制策略

从感染控制的角度来看，肺结核是最常见和最重要的疾病形式。结核病的感染防控可分为三级措施：

1. 制度管理，降低与感染性肺结核患者接触的风险；
2. 环境控制，降低感染性液滴核的浓度并防止其扩散；
3. 做好医务工作者工作期间的个人呼吸道防护。

最重要的行政措施包括及早识别潜在传染性结核病患者、及时隔离和及早开始抗结核治疗。其他措施包括对场所内的传播进行风险评估，制订感染控制计划，并培训医务人员实施该计划。必须指定一人对 IC 计划的实施进行评估和监督。

接触传染性的液滴核通常不能完全消除。因此，人们采取各种环境控制措施来降低空气中液滴核的浓度。环境措施包括通风、紫外线杀菌照射（ultraviolet germicidal irradiation，UVGI）和便携式空气净化设备。

第三个组成部分是针对性地保护医护人员，通过降低传染给它们的风险或在发生感染时降低患病风险。这些措施包括使用个人防护面罩(N95)、对医务工作者进行呼吸防护方面的培训，以及对患者进行呼吸卫生和咳嗽礼仪方面的培训[6,7]。

15.3 肺外结核

肺外结核(extrapulmonary tuberculosis，EPTB)是由结核分枝杆菌引起的感染，影响肺外的组织和器官。HIV 大流行提示了 EPTB 防控的重要性。结核病几乎可以影响我们身体的每一个器官。肺外结核最常见的形式是淋巴结结核、胃肠结核、脊柱结核和关节结核[8]。

在没有肺部或喉部受累的大多数肺外部位，结核病通常不具传染性。然而，有时冲洗结核病灶可产生感染性的液滴核，导致结核分枝杆菌的传播。当对感染的病灶进行诊断或治疗时，EPTB 可能具有传染性。

EPTB 患者可能同时患有未经确诊的肺结核或喉部结核。因此，所有患有 EPTB 的患者都应进行特定部位的检查，例如胸部 X 线片检查，痰液检测。

EPTB 的临床表现不典型，因此很难获得正确的微生物样本来确诊。但现代诊断方法(CT、MRI、腹腔镜等)为 EPTB 的诊断和定位提供了有力的支持[9]。

尽管目前的文献中缺乏结核分枝杆菌从肺外来源传播(而不是直接接种)的证据，但对 EPTB 传播的传染性和风险的深入评估在文献中并没有充分的记载[10]。

15.3.1 结核性喉炎

喉部受累通常伴有肺部受累和高度感染性。超过一半的喉结结核是血源性感染的,具有传染性。感染控制同上[6,7]。

15.3.2 气管支气管结核

气管支气管结核(tracheobronchial tuberculosis,TBTB)是指气管支气管树的结核感染,有微生物和组织病理学证据。常因非特异性症状而延误诊断。气管、支气管狭窄是 TBTB 最常见的远期并发症之一。据报道,约 10%~39%的肺结核患者合并 TBTB。对这些疾病来说,感染防控仍然是一项严峻的任务。延误诊断和非典型症状可能会增加疾病的传播率。

15.3.3 尸检中的肺结核

在尸检中,结核病并不多见(每 300 例尸检中约有 1 例),但它所带来的职业风险仍然是普通公众的 100~200 倍[11]。

感染控制策略包括:
- 尸检室合理的设计和通风
- 个人防护设备的选择
- 死者的风险评估
- 例行消毒和净化
- 使用各种方法最大限度地减少感染性气溶胶的产生
- 监测医务人员的健康

为了预防皮肤结核,皇家病理学家学会指南(http://www.rcpath.org)提出标准尸检服装和手套的建议(由乳胶和氯丁橡胶制成的双层防切割手套),以及对标准预防措施的监测。

15.3.4 脊柱结核

骨结核占所有肺外结核的 10%~20%,其中 50%~60%的骨结核病例波及脊柱。50%～75%的骨关节结核患者和高达50%的脊柱结核患者有原发性肺部病灶或有肺结核病史。

文献中共报告29例肺结核合并脊柱结核的个案。在痰抗酸杆菌涂片阴性的患者中，也出现过肺结核的呼吸道传播。一项研究发现，肺外结核患者增加了肺结核的传播率，这提示肺外结核的传染性曾被低估[12]。

CDC建议"对诊断为EPTB的患者应评估是否并发肺结核"；然而，对评估范围缺乏进一步描述。根据Mandel的传染病原理和实践，波特病（脊柱结核）患者应该常规进行胸部X线片检查，因为早期发现异常的X线片，对预后有重要影响[6]。

对疑似肺结核患者（包括脊柱结核）应进行呼吸道隔离，直到获得胸片和痰涂片和培养结果。尽管有文献报道痰涂阴性的肺结核也可传播，但往往痰涂片阴性，就会解除隔离。

对活动性肺结核采取积极的隔离措施并记录可以最大限度地减少医护人员与患者、潜在感染者的接触。

总之，结核分枝杆菌引起的疾病传播和暴发仍是巨大的挑战。为了解决这一问题，世界各地应加强结核病感染防控措施，特别是在资源有限的国家和结核病、HIV高流行的国家[13,14]。

参考文献

［1］ World Health Organization. WHO policy on TB infection control in health-care facilities, congregate settings and households. Geneva: World Health Organization; 2009.
［2］ Zumla A, Raviglione M, Hafner R, Reyn C. Tuberculosis-current perspectives. N Engl J Med. 2013; 368: 745-755.
［3］ Sterling TR, Haas DW. Transmission of mycobacterium tuberculosis from health care workers. N Engl J Med. 2006; 29: 1-4.
［4］ Pfyffer G, Palicova F. Mycobacterium: general characteristics, laboratory detection, and staining procedures. In: Versalovic J, Carroll K, Funke G, Jorgensen J, Landry M, Warnock D, editors. Manual of clinical microbiology. 10th ed. Washington, DC: ASM Press; 2011. p. 472-502.
［5］ Jarwis W. Mycobacterium tuberculosis. In: Mayhall G, editor. Hospital epidemiology and infection control. 4th ed. Philadelphia: Lippincott Williams & Wilkins; 2012.
［6］ Jensen PA, Lambert LA, Iademarco MF, et al. Guidelines for preventing the transmission of Mycobacterium tuberculosis in health-care settings, 2005.

MMWR Recomm Rep. 2005; 54(RR-17): 1-141.
[7] Menzies D, Khan FA. Nosocomial tuberculosis. In: Bennett & Brachman's hospital infections. 6th ed. Philadelphia: Lippincott Williams & Wilkins; 2014.
[8] Ramírez-Lapausa M, Menéndez-Saldaña A, Noguerado-Asensio A. Extrapulmonary tuberculosis: an overview. Rev Esp Sanid Penit. 2015; 17: 3-11.
[9] Small PM, Pai M. Tuberculosis diagnosis — time for a game change. N Engl J Med. 2010; 363(11): 1070-1071.
[10] de Vries G, Sebek MM, Lambregts-van Weezenbeek CS. Healthcare workers with tuberculosis infected during work. Eur Respir J. 2006; 28(6): 1216-1221.
[11] Flavin RJ, Gibbons N, O'Briain DS. Mycobacterium tuberculosis at autopsy — exposure and protection: an old adversary revisited. J Clin Pathol. 2007; 60(5): 487-491.
[12] Schirmer P, Renault C, Holodniy M. Is spinal tuberculosis contagious? Int J Infect Dis. 2010; 14: 659-666.
[13] Welbel SF, French AL, Bush P, et al. Protecting health care workers from tuberculosis: a 10-year experience. Am J Infect Control. 2009; 37(8): 668-673.
[14] Joshi R, Reingold AL, Menzies D, et al. Tuberculosis among health-care workers in low- and middle-income countries: a systematic review. PLoS Med. 2006; 3(12): e494.

16
重症监护病房中的肺结核

许利亚·松古尔泰金

16.1 简介

结核病是世界上最致命的疾病之一。2015年,全世界有1 000万人感染结核病,180万人死于结核病[1]。尽管结核病发病率的趋势在过去几年稳步下降,但特殊群体,包括无家可归者、囚犯、吸毒者和外国出生者,风险最高,获得医疗保障的机会最少。在土耳其,2015年共报告了12 772例肺结核病例[2]。

结核病患者入住重症监护病房(ICU)的概率从1‰~3‰[3,4]。及时诊断结核病至关重要,因为延误治疗常造成疾病加重,需入住重症监护病房。因此,了解结核的典型分布、形态和影像学表现对于重症监护医师来说是非常重要的。在ICU人群中观察到的结核发病率明显高于一般人群。大多数肺结核患者在ICU出现耐多药结核而结束了生命。这些患者患有肺结核和(或)粟粒型肺结核,并伴有严重的并发症。

16.2 ICU中的结核病表现

肺结核的临床表现包括孤立性肺结核、肺和肺外结核、孤立性肺外结核。据近期报道,在需要重症监护的重症结核病患者中,71.8%为孤立性肺结核,20.5%累及肺和肺外器官(泌尿生殖、腹膜、脑膜、淋巴、胸膜、肾和血液),7.7%为孤立性肺外结核(心包、脑膜和淋巴管)[4]。

需要ICU治疗的重症结核病通常表现为呼吸衰竭,病死率15.5%~65.9%[3,5-7]。与肺结核相关的呼吸衰竭可能与急性疾病一起发生,如粟粒型肺结核、急性呼吸窘迫综合征(acute respiratory distress syndrome,

ARDS)或支气管肺炎；也可能作为疾病的后遗症缓慢发生。巴尔克马（Balkema）等人研究显示，2/3 的患者入院的主要原因是咯血引起的急性呼吸衰竭[8]。然而，他们研究中最常见的影像学表现是弥漫性支气管肺炎。大多数肺部感染是由链球菌或金黄色葡萄球菌引起。结核分枝杆菌常与肺部细菌感染相关，最常见的是肺炎链球菌感染，尤其是儿童。社区获得性肺炎组织（Community-Acquired Pneumonia Organization，CAPO）拥有一个关于成人社区获得性肺炎（community-acquired pneumonia，CAP）的多国队列研究数据库。该组织报告说，在 6 976 例 CAP 患者中，60 例（0.86%）感染了结核分枝杆菌[9]。ICU 医师可能会发现结核分枝杆菌感染的患者，这些患者患有严重的 CAP。由结核分枝杆菌感染引起的 CAP 患者如果被误诊，可能会给医护人员和患者造成严重后果。

肺结核患者需要入住 ICU 的第二个最常见的原因是严重的脓毒症/感染性休克。这些患者大多伴有多器官功能衰竭（multiple organ failure，MOF），与其他原因入住 ICU 的患者相比，他们有更高的死亡率。播散型肺结核中的兰杜兹病是一种进展迅速的脓毒症；如果不积极治疗，会导致 MOF 和免疫功能受损的患者死亡。巴黎神经学家路易斯·西奥菲尔·约瑟夫·兰杜兹（Louis Theophile Joseph Landouzy，1845—1917）首次描述了这种疾病。这种败血症过程通常发生在免疫功能低下的患者身上，但也可能发生在免疫功能正常的患者身上[10,11]。然而，必须排除其他微生物感染才能诊断结核病相关败血症休克或败血症。

一些研究报告了危重患者中 HIV/TB 的复合感染[4,12]。HIV 和 TB 的复合感染经常发生，与单纯结核相比，复合感染常导致更高的病死率与更严重的后果。这些患者通常患有非典型肺结核，由于诊断困难和获得医疗保障的机会有限，他们的治疗可能会被延误[4]。HIV 感染常引起严严重的免疫抑制，是已知的结核病危险因素[13]。呼吸衰竭是 HIV/TB 肺部感染者入院的主要原因。这些患者中大多数都有血行播散型肺结核。从血培养中发现结核分枝杆菌提示为血行播散型结核，14% 的 HIV 患者有菌血症。ICU 入院的其他原因包括严重脓毒症/感染性休克和昏迷/迟钝。正如已发表的研究所观察到的那样，结核分枝杆菌是导致 HIV 患者出现脓毒症的常见病原体[14,15]。研究表明，播散型和肺外型肺结核患者可能是一个特殊的群体，其预后较差。HIV/TB 危重患者 6 个月内的病死率很高，其危险性与 CD4 细胞计数的最低值密切相关。即使没有原发性中枢神经系统受累，神经功能障碍也与患者生存率降低有关[12]。

16.3　ICU 中结核病的诊断

　　若有可能,应通过患者标本培养来确诊结核。这些培养物不仅能诊断结核,也为药敏试验提供了检测手段。可用于结核病诊断培养的标本包括痰液、支气管肺泡灌洗液、气管和鼻胃活检、脑脊液、心包液、腹腔液、尿液、胸腔积液、淋巴结活检和血液。

　　胸部 X 线片仍然是结核病患者初步评估的首选方法。ICU 的患者几乎没有结核病特有的症状;一些研究报告说,在胸部 X 线片检查中,若有小结节或空洞,再加上病程持续时间超过 2 周,可能预示患有结核病[16]。CT 可以识别活动性肺结核。最常见的 CT 表现为 ARDS 样表现、实质结节浸润和空洞、实变、间质受累、钙化灶、毛玻璃样混浊和胸腔积液或胸膜增厚。近50%的成人结核病患者影像学提示有淋巴结病变。在肺结核的所有肺部表现中,病死率最高的是 CT 上的 ARDS 样表现(64.5%)和粟粒型肺结核(85.5%)[17]。大多数患者有胸部 X 线片表现并不典型,仅在 CT 上有异常表现。若考虑到早期诊断,CT 扫描可以大大提高活动性肺结核的诊断率。许多活动性肺结核患者被误诊、误治。

16.4　结核病患者在 ICU 的治疗

　　感染的患者应在有负压的房间隔离,并限制探视。隔离时间取决于结核杆菌的复制周期、患者的状态以及患者的并发症,如免疫低下。确诊结核病并不容易。当怀疑有结核病时,应立即开始治疗,而不必等待培养结果。此外,即使第一次培养结果为阴性,也应继续治疗,临床医师应继续收集合适的样本进行培养。

　　急性肺结核的传统治疗方法是立即进行抗结核治疗,必要时,采用机械通气。无创正压通气(noninvasive pressure support ventilation,NIPSV)和其他辅助治疗也取得了较好的疗效[18,19]。辅助性皮质激素治疗,用于脑膜或心包疾病的治疗,与结核病患者的生存率相关[20]。类固醇激素对降低包括肺结核在内的所有需要重症监护的结核病患者的死亡率是有效的。皮质类固醇可降低因急性呼吸衰竭而入住 ICU 的肺结核患者 90 天的死亡率[21]。

在继发于肺结核的急性或慢性呼吸衰竭的情况下，患者可能需要呼吸机支持。体外膜氧合（extracorporeal membrane oxygenation，ECMO）在几种情况下对于维持不可逆心肺衰竭患者的氧合和灌流是有用的。对于肺结核患者，ECMO 对治疗难治性休克、肾功能衰竭、肝功能不全和急性呼吸窘迫综合征有效[11]。另外，在选定的患者中，在紧急情况下谨慎使用无创通气（noninvasive ventilation，NIV）可减少有创通气的使用。然而，在急性情况下使用 NIV 会增加结核病潜在传播的风险[18,22]。重症监护医师必须仔细权衡潜在的风险和益处，再决定是否启动 NIV 或有创通气治疗肺结核所致的急性呼吸衰竭。还应考虑与正压通气相关的风险，如咯血和气胸[22]。

16.5　ICU 中的结核病结局和死亡率

需要 ICU 治疗的活动性肺结核通常表现为呼吸衰竭，需要机械通气。尽管有有效的治疗方法，ICU 中结核病患者的病死率仍然在 15.5%～65.9%[3,5-7]。这个比率是 CAP 所致呼吸衰竭患者的 2 倍以上[9]。

几项研究表明，开始抗结核治疗时间越晚患者病死率越高[8]。据报道，住院治疗延迟 3～4 天，将有 33% 的肺结核患者死于急性呼吸衰竭。存活组患者从入住 ICU 到开始服用抗结核药物的间隔时间比死亡组短[23]。

ICU 病死率与年龄、机械通气、MOF、ARDS、败血症、血管活性药物使用、肾替代治疗、格拉斯哥评分低、高简化急性生理评分（SAPS II）、高序贯器官衰竭评分（SOFA）、淋巴细胞减少、低蛋白血症、低人血清白蛋白水平和两种伴随的非结核感染显著相关[3,6-9]。任何器官的衰竭都会对结核病的预后产生不良影响，且会增加病死率。然而，在所有潜在的器官功能障碍中，即使排除了原发性中枢神经系统受损的患者，死亡患者的神经功能障碍发生率也高于幸存者[6]。HIV 阳性并不是死亡的危险因素；最近的一项研究报告了 HIV/TB 复合感染患者 ICU 生存率升高的趋势[6]。在 HIV/TB 混合感染的患者中，只有 CD4 计数<200 细胞/mm³ 和没有肺叶实变与 ICU 病死率有关。

一些研究评估了肺结核患者的预后，根据肺部影像学表现的类型进行分层。他们发现，在所有肺部表现中，粟粒型肺结核（85.5%）和急性呼吸窘迫综合征（64.5%）患者的死亡率最高[17]。

总而言之，与结核病患者死亡风险相关的大多数因素都与器官衰竭的严重程度有关。其他死亡风险因素（如医院感染）实际上与重症监护过程有关。管理结核病的临床措施应以早期诊断和治疗为目标。早期诊断结核病有助于改善预后、切断传播途径。

参考文献

[1] Centers for Disease Control and Prevention (CDC). Tuberculosis. Data and Statistics. http://www.cdc.gov/tb/statistics/. Accessed 5 June 2017.
[2] WHO, Global tuberculosis report 2016. http://www.who.int/tb/publications/global_report/en/. Accessed 5 June 2017.
[3] Erbes R, Oettel K, Raffenberg M, Mauch H, Schmidt-Ioanas M, Lode H. Characteristics and outcome of patients with active pulmonary tuberculosis requiring intensive care. Eur Respir J. 2006; 27(6): 1223-1228.
[4] Duro RP, Figueiredo Dias P, Ferreira AA, Xerinda SM, Lima Alves C, Sarmento AC, Dos Santos LC. Severe tuberculosis requiring intensive care: a descriptive analysis. Crit Care Res Pract. 2017; 2017: 9535463, 9 pages.
[5] Pablos-M'endez A, Sterling TR, Frieden TR. The relationship between delayed or incomplete treatment and all-cause mortality in patients with tuberculosis. J Am Med Assoc. 1996; 276(15): 1223-1228.
[6] Lanoix J-P, Gaudry S, Flicoteaux R, Ruimy R, Wolff M. Tuberculosis in the intensive care unit: a descriptive analysis in a low-burden country. Int J Tuberc Lung Dis. 2014; 18(5): 581-587.
[7] Ryu YJ, Koh WJ, Kang EH, Suh GY, Chung MP, Kim H, Kwon OJ. Prognostic factors in pulmonary tuberculosis requiring mechanical ventilation for acute respiratory failure. Respirology. 2007; 12(3): 406-411.
[8] Balkema CA, Irusen EM, Taljaard JJ, Koegelenberg CFN. Tuberculosis in the intensive care unit: a prospective observational study. Int J Tuberc Lung Dis. 2014; 18(7): 824-830.
[9] Cavallazzi R, Wiemken T, Christensen D, Peyrani P, Blasi F, Levy G, Aliberti S, Kelley R, Ramirez J, Community-Acquired Pneumonia Organization (CAPO) Investigators. Predicting Mycobacterium tuberculosis in patients with community-acquired pneumonia. Eur Respir J. 2014; 43(1): 178-184.
[10] Geiss HK, Feldhues R, Niemann S, Nolte O, Rieker R. Landouzy septicemia (sepsis tuberculosa acutissima) due to Mycobacterium microti in an immunocompetent man. Infection. 2005; 33(5-6): 393-396.
[11] Chakravarty C, Burman S. VA-ECMO in Landouzy sepsis or tubercular septic shock. J Anesth Crit Care Open Access. 2017; 8(1): 00289.
[12] Pecego AC, Amancio RT, Ribeiro C, Mesquita EC, Medeiros DM, Cerbino J, Grinsztejn B, Bozza FA, Japiassu AM. Six-month survival of critically ill patients with HIV-related disease and tuberculosis: a retrospective study. BMC Infect Dis. 2016; 16: 270.

[13] Gary J, Cohn D. Tuberculosis and HIV Coinfection. Semin Respir Crit Care Med. 2013; 34(01): 032-43.

[14] Japiassú AM, Amancio RT, Mesquita EC, Medeiros DM, Bernal HB, Nunes EP, et al. Sepsis is a major determinant of outcome in critically ill HIV/AIDS patients. Crit Care. 2010; 14(4): R152.

[15] Crump JA, Ramadhani HO, Morrissey AB, Saganda W, Mwako MS, Yang LY, et al. Bacteremic disseminated tuberculosis in sub-saharan Africa: a prospective cohort study. Clin Infect Dis. 2012; 55(2): 242-250.

[16] Hui C, Wu CL, Chan MC, Kuo IT, Chiang CD. Features of severe pneumonia in patients with undiagnosed pulmonary tuberculosis in an intensive care unit. J Formos Med Assoc. 2003; 102: 563-569.

[17] Hashemian SM, Tabarsi P, Karam MB, Kahkouee S, Marjani M, Jamaati H, Shekarchi N, Mohajerani SA, Velayati AA. Radiologic manifestations of pulmonary tuberculosis in patients of intensive care units. Int J Mycobacteriol. 2015; 4(3): 233-238.

[18] Agarwal R, Gupta D, Handa A, Aggarwal ANR. Noninvasive ventilation in ARDS caused by Mycobacterium tuberculosis: report of three cases and review of literature. Intensive Care Med. 2005; 31(12): 1723-1724.

[19] Flores-Franco RA, Olivas-Medina DA, Pacheco-Tena CF, Duque-Rodríguez J. Immunoadjuvant therapy and noninvasive ventilation for acute respiratory failure in lung tuberculosis: a case study. Case Rep Pulmonol. 2015; 2015: 283867. Epub 2015 Jul 27.

[20] Nahid P, Dorman SE, Alipanah N, Barry PM, Brozek JL, Cattamanchi A, Chaisson LH, Chaisson RE, Daley CL, Grzemska M, Higashi JM, Ho CS, Hopewell PC, Keshavjee SA, Lienhardt C, Menzies R, Merrifield C, Narita M, O'Brien R, Peloquin CA, Raftery A, Saukkonen J, Schaaf HS, Sotgiu G, Starke JR, Migliori GB, Vernon A. Official American Thoracic Society/Centers for Disease Control and Prevention/Infectious Diseases Society of America Clinical Practice Guidelines: treatment of drug-susceptible tuberculosis. Clin Infect Dis. 2016; 63(7): e147-195.

[21] Critchley JA, Young F, Orton L, Garner P. Corticosteroids for prevention of mortality in people with tuberculosis: a systematic review and meta-analysis. Lancet Infect Dis. 2013; 13(3): 223-237.

[22] Jensen PA, Lambert LA, Iademarco MF, et al. Guidelines for preventing the transmission of Mycobacterium tuberculosis in health-care settings, 2005. MMWR Recomm Rep. 2005; 54: 1-141.

[23] Levy H, Kallenbach JM, Feldman C, Thorburn JR, Abramowitz JA. Acute respiratory failure in active tuberculosis. Crit Care Med. 1987; 15: 221-225.

索引

C 反应蛋白　94,169
Erlich-Ziehl-Neelsen 染色　65,107
γ-干扰素　28,185

B

白细胞尿　144,147,149
吡嗪酰胺　11,21,49,68,75,92,112,
　113,128,129,139,150,161,180,186
波特病　9,94,135,193
布鲁里溃疡　180
布鲁氏菌病　91

C

肠结核　26-29,31-38,191
肠组织　35
纯化蛋白衍生物　65,136,167

D

大动脉炎　156,164,165,167
胆管狭窄　47
地塞米松　129,130
动脉粥样硬化　169,170
对氨基水杨酸　92
多器官衰竭　50
多灶性骨关节结核　76

F

非结核分枝杆菌　61,74,84,86,91,
　109,127,148,165,179,180
肺炎链球菌　196

氟喹诺酮类　112,129,148
腹部结核　2,4,10,26,30,44,51
腹膜结核　30,31,33
腹腔镜检查　34,46,48,53

G

感觉诱发电位　94
巩膜炎　184
骨关节结核　4,9,10,72,73,75,77,
　80,193

H

核酸扩增试验　19,66,79,111
虹膜睫状体炎　182
喉结核　4
后葡萄膜炎　182,183
霍奇金病　48

J

肌肉骨骼结核　9,91,93
肌肉骨骼系统　10,80
急性呼吸窘迫综合征　195,198
脊髓蛛网膜炎　8
脊柱感染　135
脊柱炎　76,85,88,91,136,138,
　140,164
脊椎骨髓炎　84,87
焦磷酸测序　66
结核菌素皮肤试验　36,48,65,75,109,
　160,185

结核瘤 2,8,45,90,105,113,163
结核性骶髂关节炎 76
结核性腹膜炎 26,27,30,34-38,50
结核性肝脓肿 44,46-49
结核性骨髓炎 9,72,76-80,84
结核性关节炎 72,73,77,78,84,135
结核性喉炎 192
结核性脊柱炎 9,88,89
结核性结膜炎 184
结核性淋巴结炎 4,8,10,50,60,61,68,167
结核性脑膜炎 8,50,102,103,106-108,112-114,126,127,129,130,138
结核性脑炎 124-126,128-131
结核性心包炎 50,156-162
结核性胸腔积液 2,16,19-21
结核性牙龈瘤 178
结核硬脂酸 110
结节性疾病 46
金黄色葡萄球菌 72,78,91,185,196
静脉尿路造影 144
静脉肾盂造影 148,149
静脉血栓栓塞 170
酒精性肝病 27

K

卡介苗 46,53,67,103,109,145,146,165,169,170,178
抗逆转录病毒治疗 94,113
抗酸染色 19,35,53,65,185
抗肿瘤坏死因子 176
克罗恩病 10,29,30,32,33,38

L

朗汉斯巨细胞 45,53,105
泪囊炎 184
类风湿性关节炎 20,72,76,169

利福平 7,11,21,49,66,68,75,79,80,91,92,112-114,128,129,139,150,161,170,180,186
淋巴结病 30,32,52,108,158,167,197
淋巴结核 5,62,63,65,67
淋巴结结核 2,4,7,8,29,60,61,63-68,191
淋巴结肿大 7,10,18,46,64,68
淋巴细胞减少 198
颅内结核瘤 8

M

脉络膜结节 184
脉络膜炎 182,183
酶联免疫斑点 138,161
酶联免疫吸附试验 108,137,138
泌尿生殖道结核 143
免疫抑制 2,16,19,51,60-62,72,85,86,103,109,110,114,130,178,180,186,196
免疫重建炎症综合征 21,30,94,113,130

N

耐多药结核病 92,113,139,140,150,176
耐药结核 9,21,36,37,92,113,150
男性生殖器结核 144,145
脑积水 9,102,104-106,108,109,113,114,130
脑脓肿 9,128,130
尿路结核 145,151

P

皮肤结核 4,176,177,180,192
皮质类固醇 21,113,114,158,186,197
脾结核 44,50-54

索引

葡萄膜炎 182,183,185

Q

气管支气管结核 192
丘疹坏死性结核 179

R

肉芽肿性肝炎 45,46
肉芽肿性疾病 7,91

S

沙利度胺 113,130
社区获得性肺炎 196
神经视网膜炎 184
渗出性缩窄性心包炎 157,159
生殖器结核 143,144,148
食管结核 28
视神经病变 150,184-186
缩窄性心包炎 157-162

T

吞噬体 62

W

韦格纳肉芽肿 20
胃肠道结核 10
无创通气 198

X

系统性红斑狼疮 20,51
细针抽吸 10,53,65
细针吸取细胞学 148
狭窄成形术 37
线探针分析 111
腺苷脱氨酶 19,20,34,110,127,161
小肠结核 29

心包穿刺术 159,160
心包积液 157-162
心包溶菌酶 161
心包炎 156-161,163,164
心血管结核 156
胸膜结核 17,19
胸腔积液 16-18,20,21,108,158,159,185,197
血行播散 5,50,77,108,157,162,176-178,182,196

Y

眼底荧光血管造影 186
眼眶超声 186
眼内炎 184,185
液滴核 190,191
乙胺丁醇 11,21,49,68,75,92,112,128,129,139,161,180,186,187
异烟肼 7,11,21,49,66,68,75,92,112-114,128,129,139,150,161,163,180,186,187
游泳池肉芽肿 179
鱼缸肉芽肿 179
运动诱发电位 94

Z

支气管肺炎 196
中枢神经系统 2,9,102,105,111,112,124,129,156,183,196,198
中枢神经系统结核 2,8,11,103,108,110,127
肿瘤坏死因子 17,28,109,157,169
主动脉炎和动脉瘤 164
转移性结核性脓肿 178
纵隔淋巴结病 160